# Creepy Crawlies

Written by John Stidworthy
Illustrated by Michael Posen

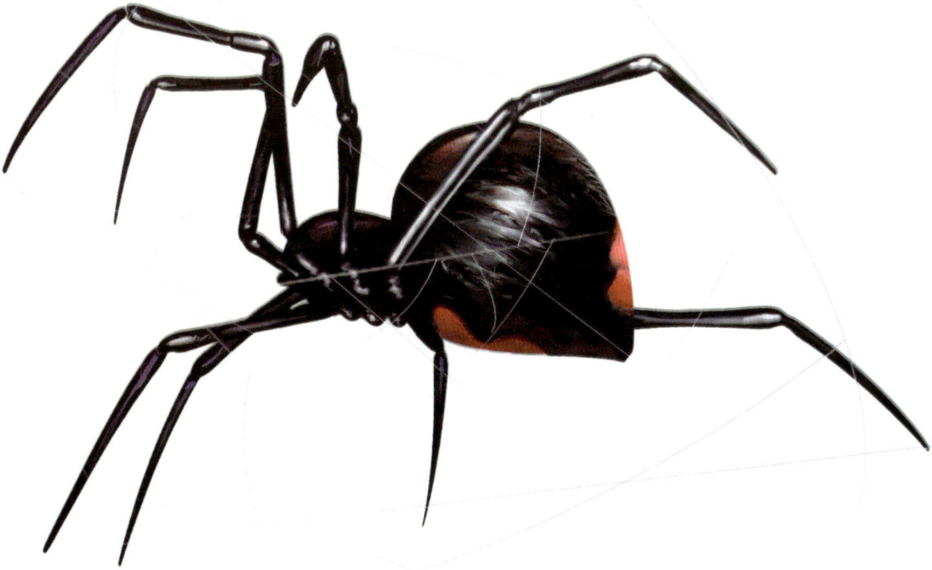

p

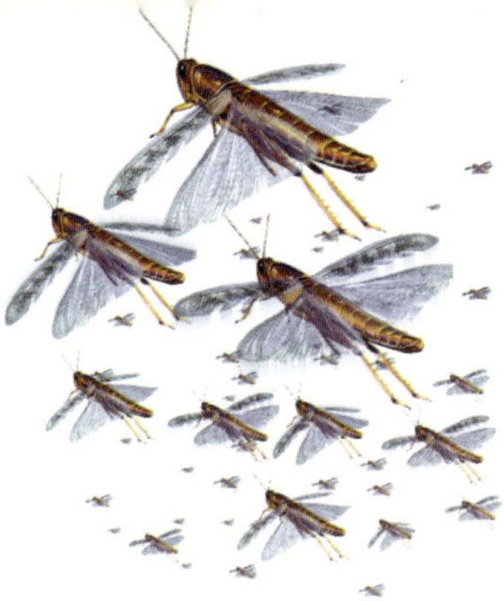

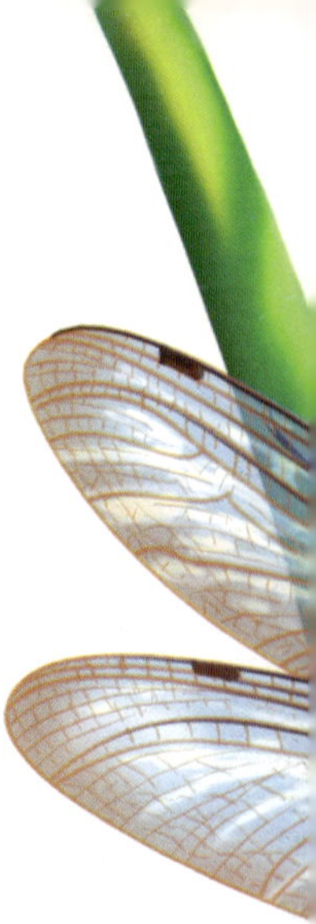

This is a Parragon Publishing Book
This edition published in 2002

Parragon Publishing
Queen Street House
4 Queen Street
Bath BA1 1HE, UK



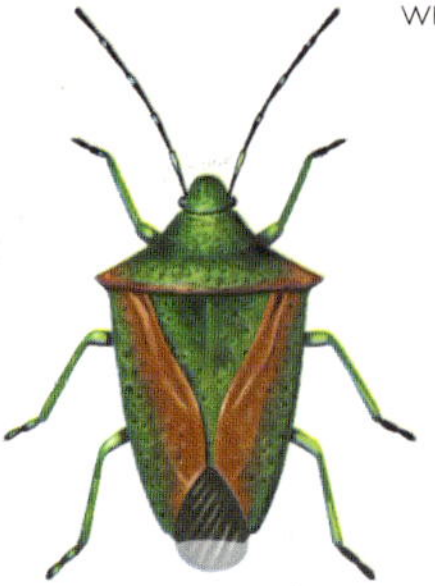

ISBN 0-75259-652-7

Printed in China

Produced by
Monkey Puzzle Media Ltd

Cover design: Design Principals

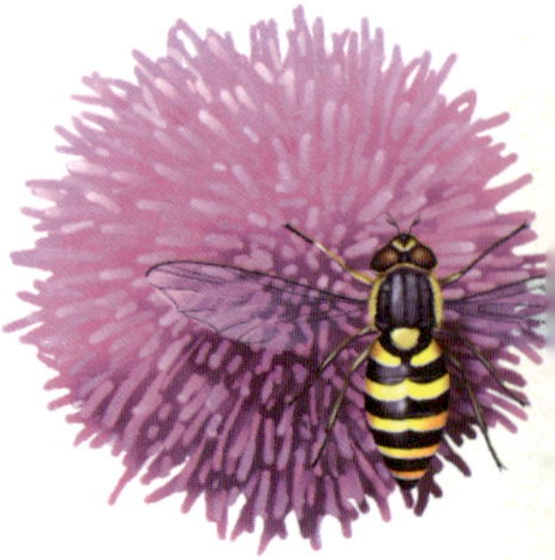

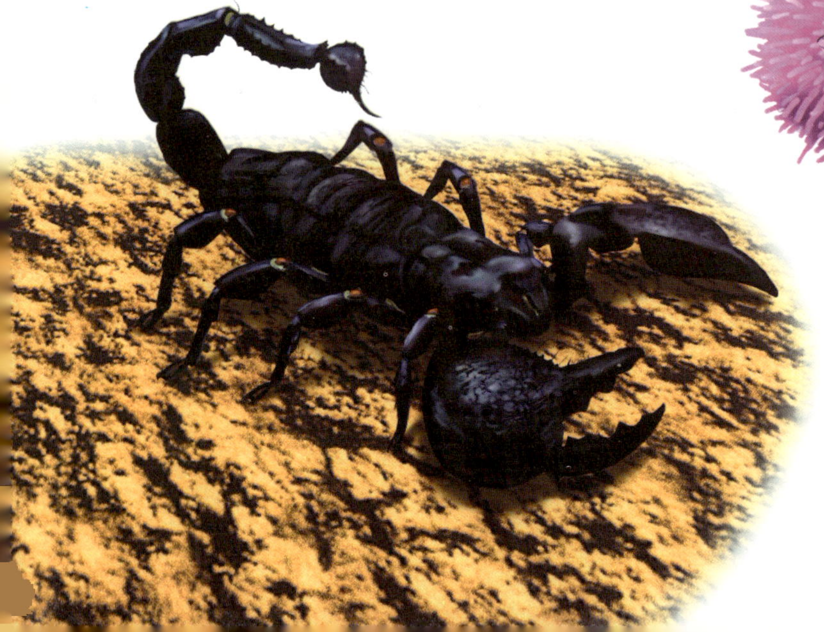

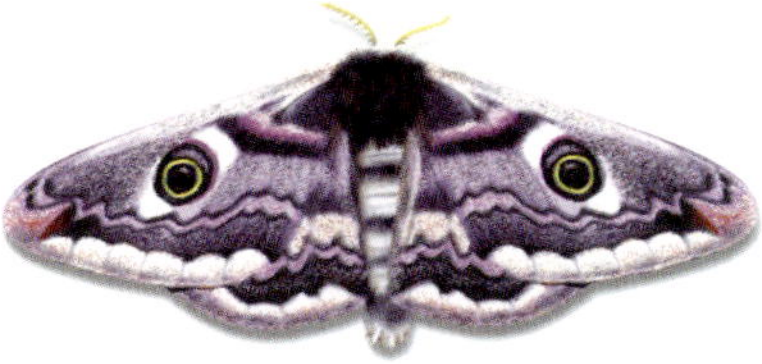

# Contents

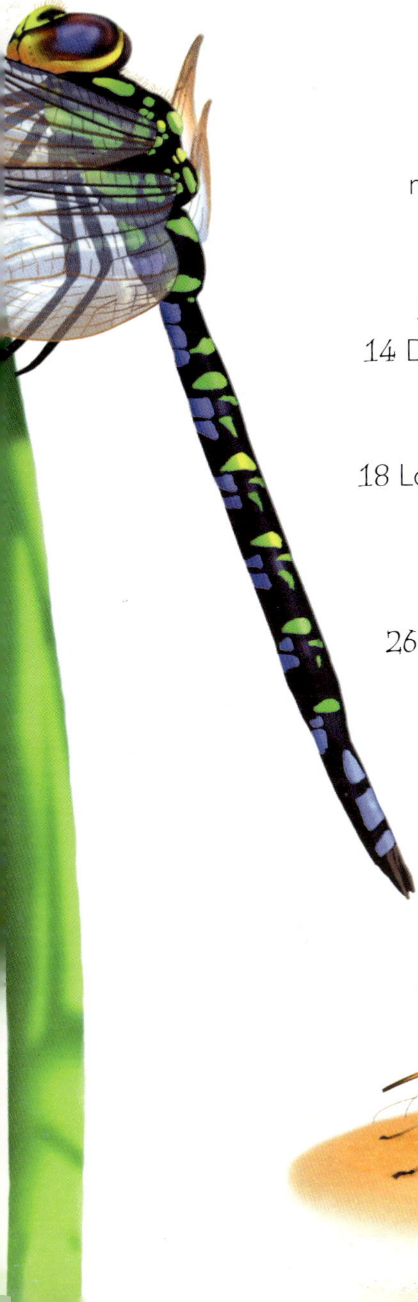


4 Spiders
6 Scorpions, ticks, mites, and millipedes
8 Termites
10 Ants
12 Bees and wasps
14 Dragonflies, mantids, and stick insects
16 Bugs
18 Locusts and grasshoppers
20 Fleas and lice
22 Flies
24 Beetles
26 Butterflies and moths
28 Worms
30 Slugs and snails
32 Index


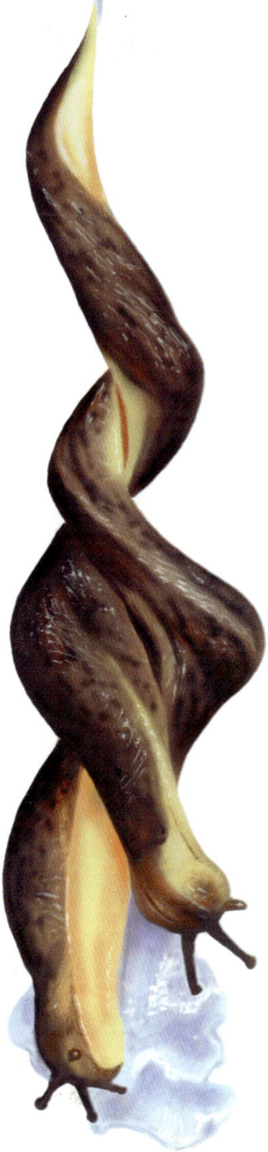

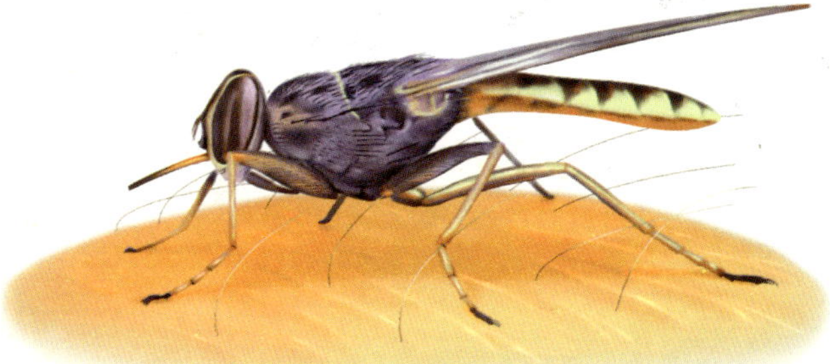

# Which are the biggest spiders?

THE "BIRD-EATING" SPIDERS OF SOUTH AMERICA ARE BOTH THE HEAVIEST and widest species, with weights up to 3 oz (80 g) and leg spans up to 10 in (26 cm). Very few of them actually eat birds, but the bigger species do eat small frogs, lizards, and snakes.

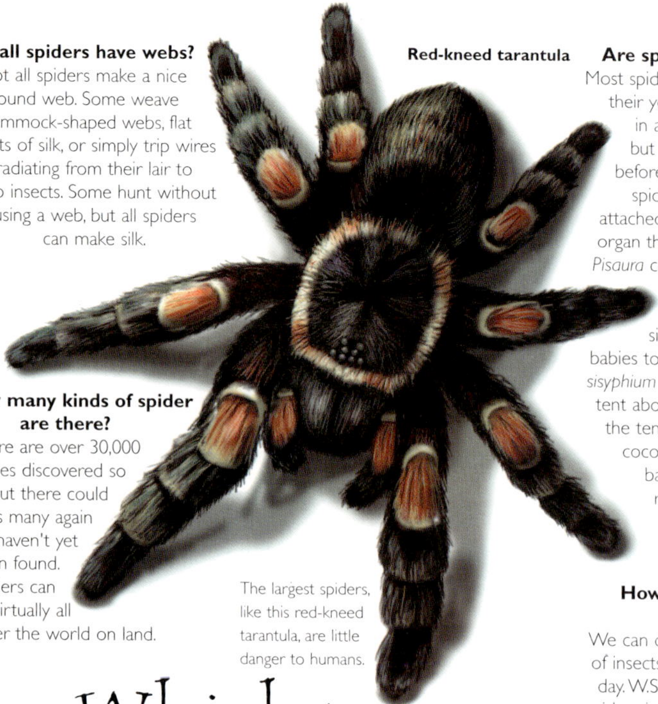

Red-kneed tarantula

The largest spiders, like this red-kneed tarantula, are little danger to humans.

**Do all spiders have webs?**
Not all spiders make a nice round web. Some weave hammock-shaped webs, flat sheets of silk, or simply trip wires radiating from their lair to trap insects. Some hunt without using a web, but all spiders can make silk.

**How many kinds of spider are there?**
There are over 30,000 species discovered so far, but there could be as many again that haven't yet been found. Spiders can live virtually all over the world on land.

**Which spider makes the biggest webs?**
The tropical orb web spiders can have webs over 16 ft (5 m) across. Up to 2,300 ft (700 m) length of silk strand can be produced by the silk glands of one of these spiders. The silk is so strong it can actually hold a human.

Crab spider

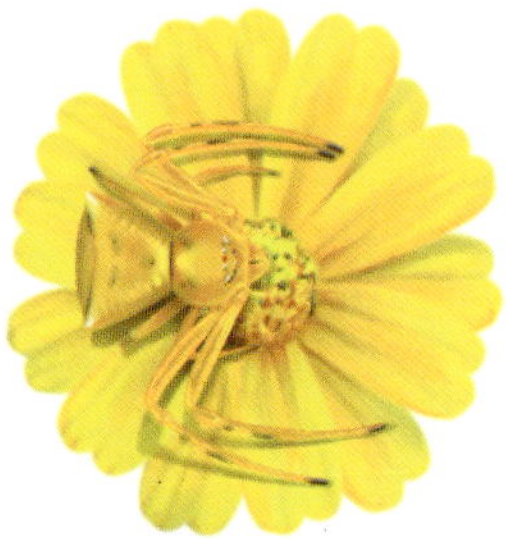

A crab spider can change color to match the flower it is on.

**Are spiders good parents?**
Most spiders don't really look after their young. Many lay their eggs in a cocoon, for protection, but often the female will die before they hatch. Mother wolf spiders carry the cocoon attached to their spinnerets (the organ that makes their silk), and *Pisaura* carries her cocoon in her fangs until hatching time, when she builds a silk tent, on a plant, for the babies to live in. The tiny *Theridion sisyphium* lives in a thimble-shaped tent above its hammock web. In the tent it looks after the egg cocoon, then feeds the tiny babies below it with the regurgitated juices from the prey.

**How many insects do spiders eat?**
We can only guess at the millions of insects eaten by spiders every day. W.S. Bristowe, who studied spiders in England, once calculated that, over a year, spiders ate a weight of insects greater than the weight of all the people living in England.

**Why do spiders spit?**
*Scytodes*, a small black and yellow spider, found in Europe and the USA, has an unusual way of catching its prey. As an insect approaches, the spider raises its fangs and ejects two streams of gum from them, swinging its head so that the two lines of gum fall in a zigzag over the prey. Once the prey is pinned down, the spider moves in to bite and eat it.

**How many eyes does a spider have?**
Most spiders have eight eyes, but there are species with six, four or two. The shape and arrangement of the eyes help to tell which family a spider belongs to. Many spiders use touch more than sight, but the eyes of jumping spiders are well developed.

**Can spiders fly?**
Spiders do not have wings, but many species can parachute, or sail through the air by letting out a long thread of silk until they are carried away by the wind. Many young spiders leave the nest by this "ballooning" technique. They can be carried thousands of yards above the earth.

**Which spiders give presents?**
Male spiders are often smaller than their mates. Sometimes the female may attack the male in order to eat him. Many American wolf spiders "sing" to the female to distract her and try and save themselves. The male spider *Pisaura mirabilis* of Europe makes himself safe by catching a fly, wrapping it into a silk parcel, and presenting it to the female, who eats it as they mate. He does this in the hope that she won't be hungry enough to make a meal of him.

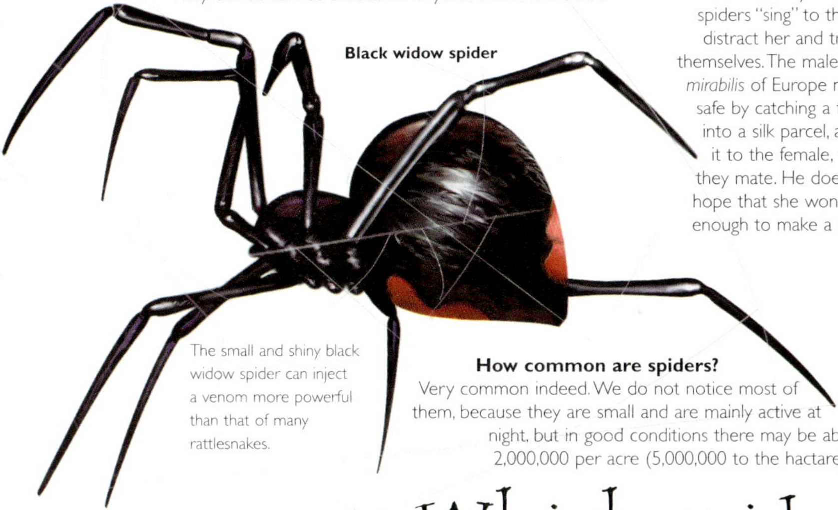

**Black widow spider**

The small and shiny black widow spider can inject a venom more powerful than that of many rattlesnakes.

**How common are spiders?**
Very common indeed. We do not notice most of them, because they are small and are mainly active at night, but in good conditions there may be about 2,000,000 per acre (5,000,000 to the hactare).

# Which spiders are human killers?

ALL SPIDERS ARE POISONOUS, BUT ONLY A FEW HAVE STRONG ENOUGH FANGS, and powerful enough venom, to harm people. The black widow, found in many warm parts of the world, including the USA and Europe, is a small, round spider which likes hiding in quiet places. It is not aggressive, but if it is attacked, it may bite. After a few minutes, the bite is terribly painful. The victim feels dizzy, and can suffer from paralysis. It is rarely fatal, though, and nowadays cures are available. The Australian Sydney funnel-web spider is a larger species with a dangerous bite. A bite from this spider causes heart failure and breathing problems. Again, drugs are now available to reverse the effects. The recluse spiders of the USA, and the Brazilian wandering spider, have bites that can be fatal. However, the chances of being killed by a spider are less than those of being struck by lightning.

**Can spiders change color?**
The crab spiders, such as *Misumena*, live in flowers. They lie in wait for insects, sitting on flowers whose colors they match. They are even capable of changing color over a few days to match the flower. Most kinds of spider stay the same color, but their natural coloring or pattern is often perfect camouflage for their habitat.

**Which spider likes to go fishing?**
The bolas spider hangs underneath a branch on a silky trapeze, then lets down a silk line about 2 in (5 cm) long with a sticky blob on the end. The spider swings this around to catch passing insects.

**What is a spider's web made of?**
A spider's web is made of silk. Spiders have glands on their abdomen which produce the silk, which can be made sticky, elastic or very strong. Some spider silk is much stronger than steel of the same thickness.

# When do scorpions dance?

THE MATING RITUAL OF SCORPIONS LOOKS LIKE A DANCE. THE partners grab one another's pincers, to protect themselves from each other. With pincers held, they move back, forward and sideways, sometimes for hours. Finally, the male deposits a packet of sperm and moves the female over on top of it. The sperm goes into her body and fertilizes the eggs.

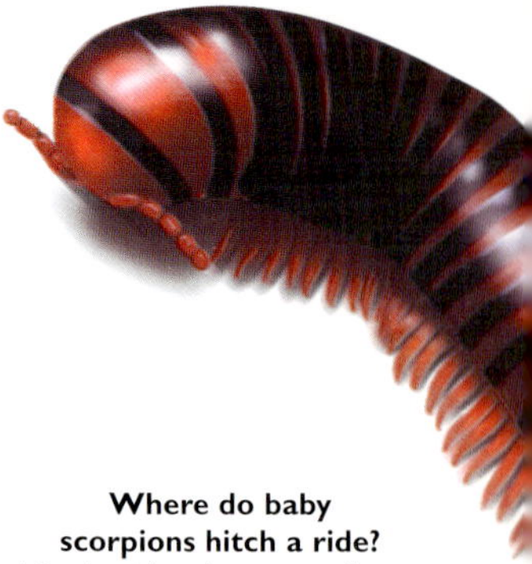

**Where do baby scorpions hitch a ride?**
After hatching, the young of many scorpions climb onto their mother's back. They use her large pincers as a climbing ramp. They ride there until after their first molt (when they lose a layer of skin). After this they leave their mother and start to fend for themselves.

**Where do the biggest scorpions live?**
The largest scorpions live in tropical forests. Some, such as the imperial scorpion of Africa, are up to 7 in (18 cm) long. These scorpions aren't very poisonous.

**Do all scorpions sting?**
All scorpions have poisonous stings at the ends of their tails. They use them mainly to defend themselves. Only a few are truly dangerous to humans. Most scorpion stings are unpleasant, rather than deadly.

**Why do ticks drink blood?**
Ticks don't find food very often, and they must be ready to latch on to anything that can provide it, as it passes. An adult tick may have to wait months, or even years, before fastening its jaws into a passing mammal and sucking its blood. It has to have a meal of blood before it can lay its eggs.

Scorpions first appeared on earth 345 million years ago.

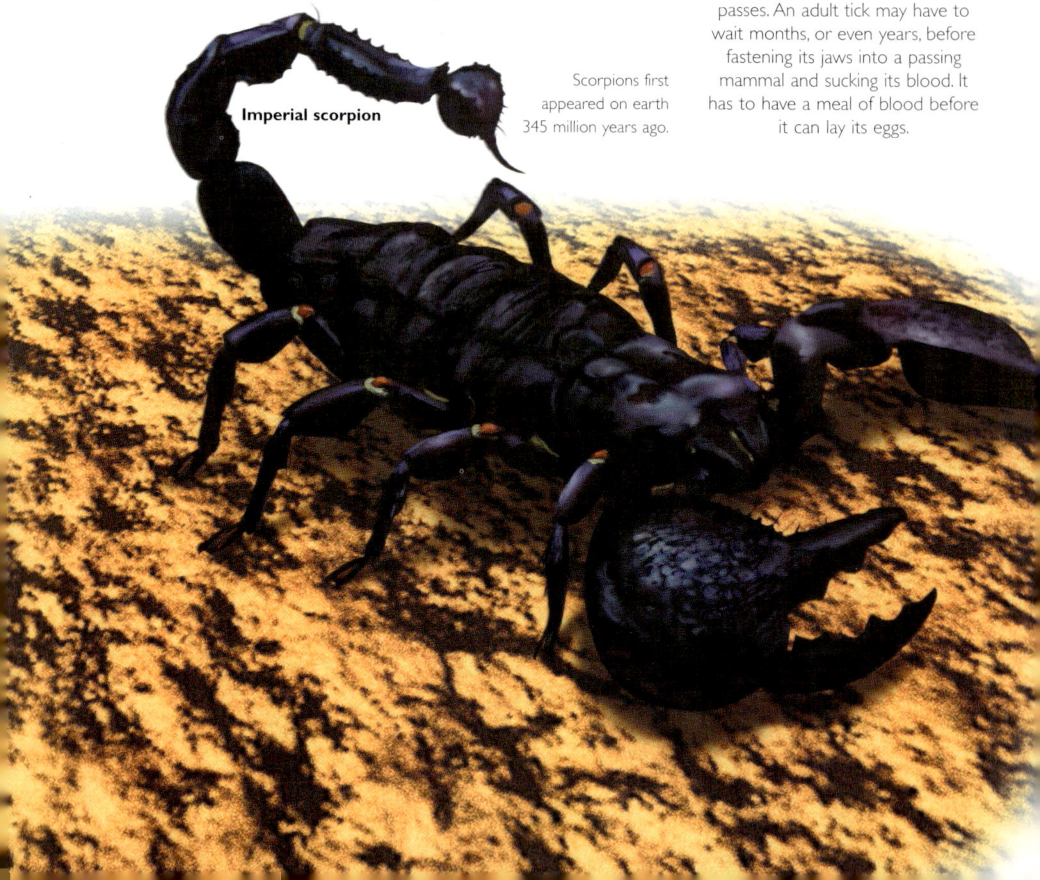

**Imperial scorpion**

### How many legs does a millipede really have?

In spite of their name (*mille* is Latin for a thousand), millipedes never have a thousand legs. The most that they have is 200 pairs (400 legs), and some species have only 20 pairs (40 legs). The leg movements are co-ordinated in "waves" running from front to back.

### Will you ever be attacked by a centipede?

Centipedes have a pair of poison fangs, that they use to catch their prey. Most centipedes in countries with a mild climate, do not have a powerful enough bite to do serious damage. Anyway, they usually run away rather than attack. But some large tropical centipedes can inflict a nasty bite if threatened.

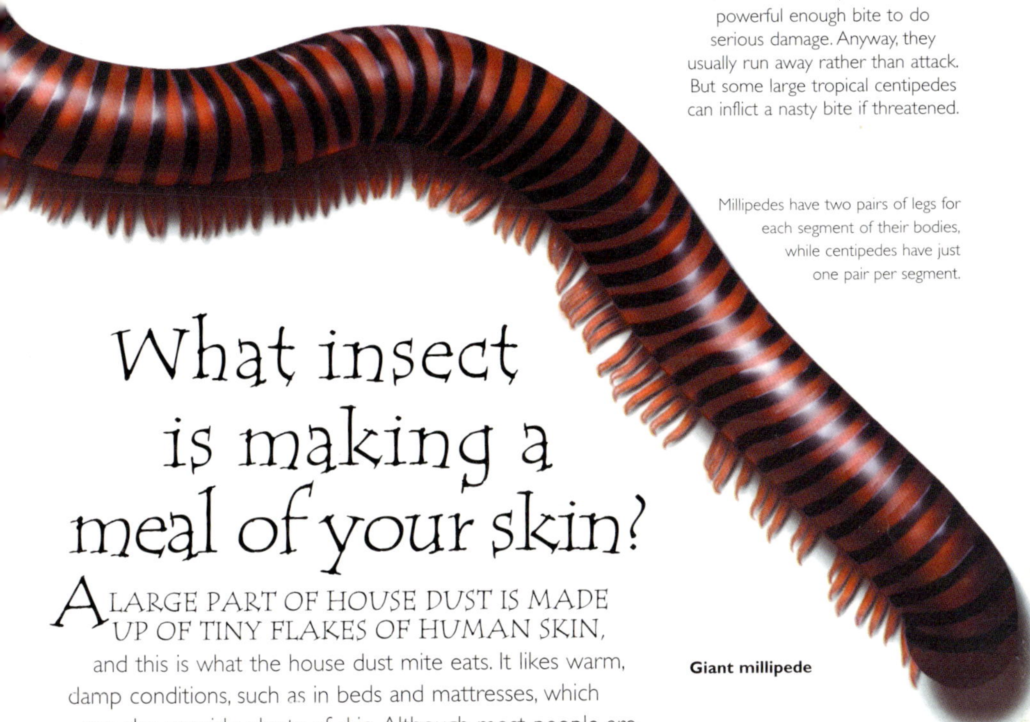

Millipedes have two pairs of legs for each segment of their bodies, while centipedes have just one pair per segment.

**Giant millipede**

# What insect is making a meal of your skin?

A LARGE PART OF HOUSE DUST IS MADE UP OF TINY FLAKES OF HUMAN SKIN, and this is what the house dust mite eats. It likes warm, damp conditions, such as in beds and mattresses, which can also provide plenty of skin. Although most people are not affected by these mites, some people are highly allergic to them.

### How can you tell a millipede from a centipede?

Most millipedes are slow-moving plant-eaters with short legs and chewing mouthparts. Centipedes are fast-moving meat-eaters with fangs that they use to kill prey. They have fewer legs than millipedes.

### What animal lives in your eyelashes?

Almost all of us have tiny mites living in the sockets of our eyes. They do no harm and may even help to keep our skin clean. They are so small that we can't see them.

### What do centipedes have for dinner?

Centipedes eat insects, slugs, and other creepy-crawlies; they even eat other centipedes. The largest tropical species can be 13 in (33 cm) long. They can kill animals such as lizards, frogs and mice.

### How big are the biggest millipedes?

Some of the millipedes that live in the tropical parts of Africa grow to 11 in (28 cm) or more, with a diameter (thickness) of about 1 in (2 cm).

### What tick carries a mountainous disease?

A serious illness, called Rocky Mountain fever, is caused by a tiny organism called a rickettsia. It invades the cells of the body and produces severe fever. The disease is carried by woodchucks, but wood ticks, living on these animals, can carry it to humans. The disease was first discovered in Montana, about 100 years ago, when it killed three-quarters of those who got it. Since then, it has been found in other parts of North and South America, but not in such a deadly form.

# What weapons does a soldier termite have?

SOLDIER TERMITES ARE TOUGHER THAN THE WORKER TERMITES. MANY termite species have soldiers, with huge armored heads and biting jaws, to fight off enemies, particularly ants. Other species have soldiers with special "snouts" that can shoot sticky fluid over an enemy. Soldiers are designed only for fighting, so they cannot even feed themselves. They have to rely on the workers to provide food for them.

**Why are termites heavier than elephants?**

Millions of termites live in the tropics. There may be as many as 3,300 per square yard (4,000 per square metre), sometimes even twice this. The weight of termites in 0.4 square miles (1 square kilometre) under the ground, is more than the weight of all the elephants or zebras feeding on the vegetation above the ground.

**Which insect likes a termite bite?**

Termites are a tasty food to other insects, particularly ants. Many birds also eat them. There are also many mammals, that are equipped with sharp claws, to break into termite nests, and long tongues to lap the termites up. These include: the South American tamanduas and giant "anteaters," the aardvark of Africa, and pangolins in Africa and Asia.

**What's the difference between a termite and an ant?**

There isn't a lot of difference between them, ants eat other creatures, but termites like to stick to plants. Although termites are sometimes called "white ants," they are much more like cockroaches than ants. Termites have been around for millions of years, and are great recyclers of plant materials.

**What is a termite garden?**

Some species of termite, including *Macrotermes*, farm, or grow, a fungus. They make special "fungus combs" out of their own faeces, as a base on which to grow the fungus. These are called "gardens." The fungus breaks down the faeces, and the termites feed on the fungus, and its products. The fungus is a special one, only found growing in termite nests.

**Who helps termites digest their food?**

Wood-eating termites do not actually digest wood themselves, but rely on protozoa (single-celled animals) that live in their gut to break it down. In the gut of other termites, large colonies of bacteria help to break down food. Termites also contain bacteria that take nitrogen from the air and turn it into body-building protein. Termites owe their success to these tiny creatures in their guts.

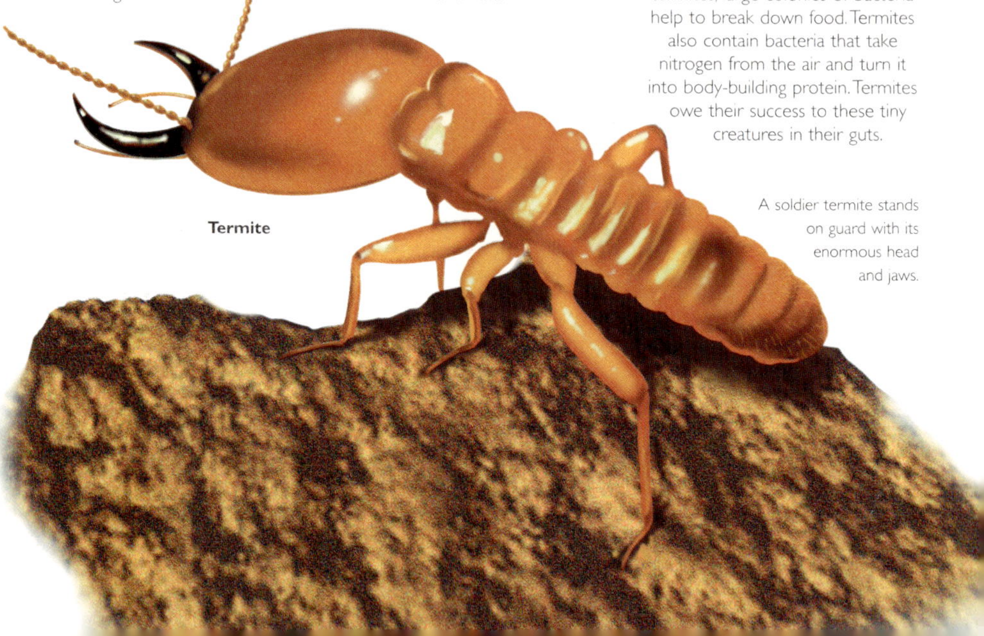

**Termite**

A soldier termite stands on guard with its enormous head and jaws.

**Why are some termites magnetic?**

Magnetic termites live in Australia. They build a nest in a flat blade shape. The flat sides point east and west, catching the cooler morning and evening sun, but only the narrow edge points north to the midday sun, so that only a little of the nest catches the sun at its hottest. The nest is often used as a compass by people in the bush, and this is how the nest gets its name.

**Which insects have air-conditioned nests?**

In insect nests, most of the "living accommodation" is below ground. So, in hot climates, they could overheat. Termites such as *Macrotermes* build a hollow nest with a central chimney and side channels to allow the circulation of air. Wind blowing across the top of the tall chimney helps to draw out air and create a breeze.

**Termite mound**

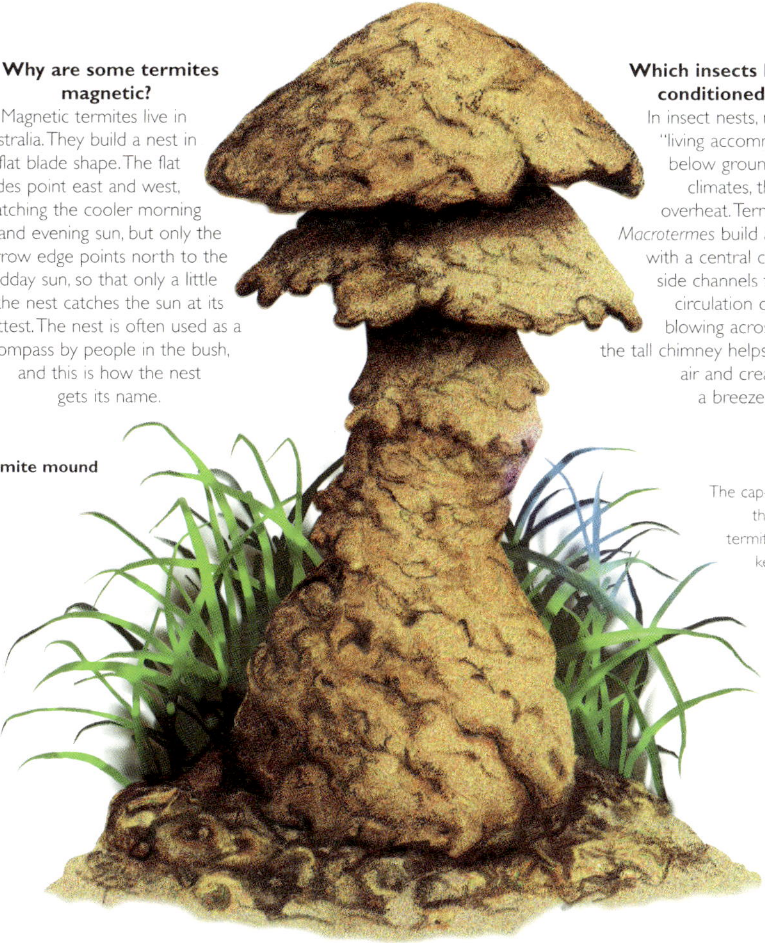

The cap-shaped roof, of this African forest termite mound, helps keep off the rain.

# What is a termite city?

A NUMBER OF TERMITES IN THE TROPICAL DRY SAVANNAS BUILD VERY HIGH mounds. These are where termites live and work. Some of them are very big. The magnetic termite mounds can be 11 ft (3.5 m) tall. In Africa, *Macrotermes* builds nests that can extend up to 24 ft (7.5 m), four times the height of a human. In contrast, some species make their nests entirely within one plant, or underground and they are quite small.

**How many eggs does a queen termite lay?**

The queen termite's only job is to lay eggs, and she may become much bigger than her surrounding workers, when her huge abdomen is filled with eggs. In some species, the queen lays up to 30,000 eggs a day.

**Which termites are suicide bombers?**

There are termite species which don't have a soldier caste. The workers defend the nest from attackers. If ants attack the colony, the workers burst their guts open, throwing the slimy contents over the enemy, and killing themselves at the same time.

# How do ants defend their nests?

MANY KINDS OF ANT ARE ARMED WITH STINGS FOR PROTECTION. OTHERS, such as the big wood ant of Europe, can squirt formic acid at enemies. Species with large soldier ants may rely on their jaws to attack invaders. Some species have more specialized ways of keeping trouble out, such as soldiers that block the entrance to the nest with their body.

**When is an ant like a honeypot?**
Among *Myrmecocystus* ants, of North America, some of the workers are actually used as storage jars. They never go out of the nest, and are fed the spare nectar gathered by workers. Their abdomens swell massively as they become living stores, to be called on when food is short.

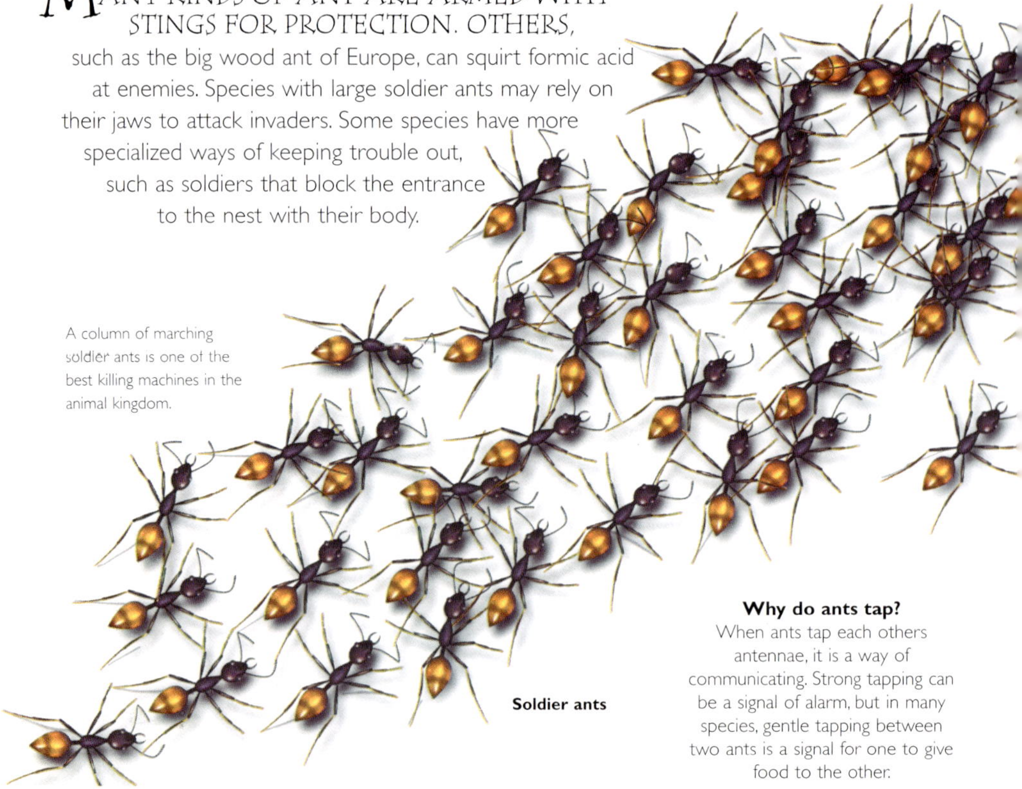

A column of marching soldier ants is one of the best killing machines in the animal kingdom.

**Soldier ants**

**Why do ants tap?**
When ants tap each others antennae, it is a way of communicating. Strong tapping can be a signal of alarm, but in many species, gentle tapping between two ants is a signal for one to give food to the other.

**Which ants like a thorny home?**
The acacia ant makes its small nest just in the spiny tips of twigs of acacia thorn trees, in the Savanna (dry plains with bushes and trees). The ants get some protection from the thorns, and they keep the tree free of other, harmful insects by eating them.

**How do ants grow mushrooms?**
The leaf-cutter ants, of tropical America, cut out pieces of leaf to take back to their nest and use as a kind of "manure." Back in their nests, underground, they chew the leaves and add them to their "garden." A fungus grows in this garden (each ant species has its own) which makes a nutritious food.

**Why do ants need slaves?**
Some ants are forced to act as workers for other species. The slave-maker ant, of Europe, raids the nests of other species and carries the young back to their own nest. When they hatch out, these new workers act as slaves collecting food, feeding other ants, and cleaning the nest. Slavery is used by a few ant species.

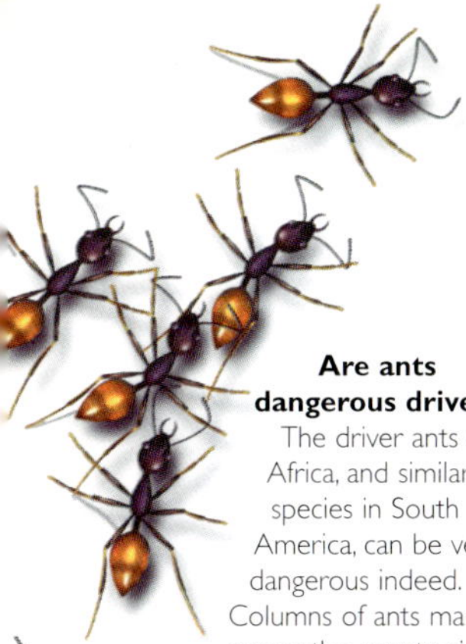

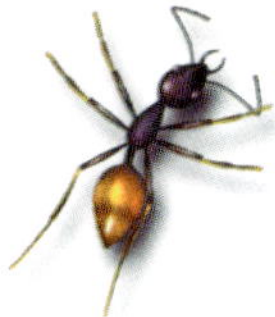

**Are ants dangerous drivers?**
The driver ants of Africa, and similar species in South America, can be very dangerous indeed. Columns of ants march across the countryside, attacking and eating everything that cannot escape. Animals, from insects to snakes, and even humans, may be attacked by thousands of ferocious ants.

**Why do ants have wings?**
Ants' wings are only used when they mate. Only fully-grown males and females have wings. Workers do not need them. When they land from their mating flights, females that have been fertilized lose their wings, in some cases chewing them off. They then look for a place to start a new colony and have their young.

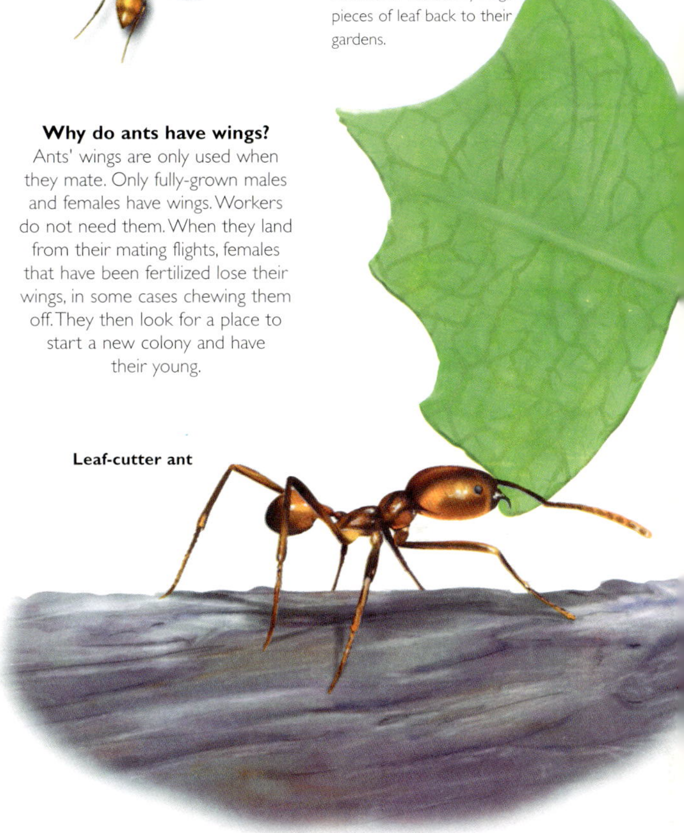

Leaf-cutter ants carry huge pieces of leaf back to their gardens.

**Leaf-cutter ant**

**Which ants look after "cows"?**
Several kinds of ant feed on a sweet substance, called honeydew, which is produced by aphids (a small bug, such as a greenfly). Some, like the black garden ant, look after herds of aphid "cows" or females, protecting them from predators, and even moving them to new plants on which to feed.

**Are all ants sociable?**
All ant species are social animals. This means that they live in groups and each of them is given a job to do in the colony. Each colony has at least one egg-laying female, or queen, but she is vastly outnumbered by the ants we usually see, the workers. They are wingless and sterile females – never males.

**How many ants are there in an ant nest?**
Some estimates put the number of ants in such a nest as high as 7 million. Other species have smaller nests, with numbers ranging from thousands to hundreds. The biggest ant nests are those made by the leaf-cutter ants, some of which travel for 33 ft (10 m) or more underground.

# How do ants know each other?

ANTS PROBABLY DON'T RECOGNIZE EACH OTHER AS INDIVIDUALS. BUT EACH species has its own chemical messengers, and there may be slight differences between nests too. An ant can recognize another as a nest mate, or a stranger, by its smell. Chemicals allow the ants to leave scent trails that can be followed by others to good food sources.

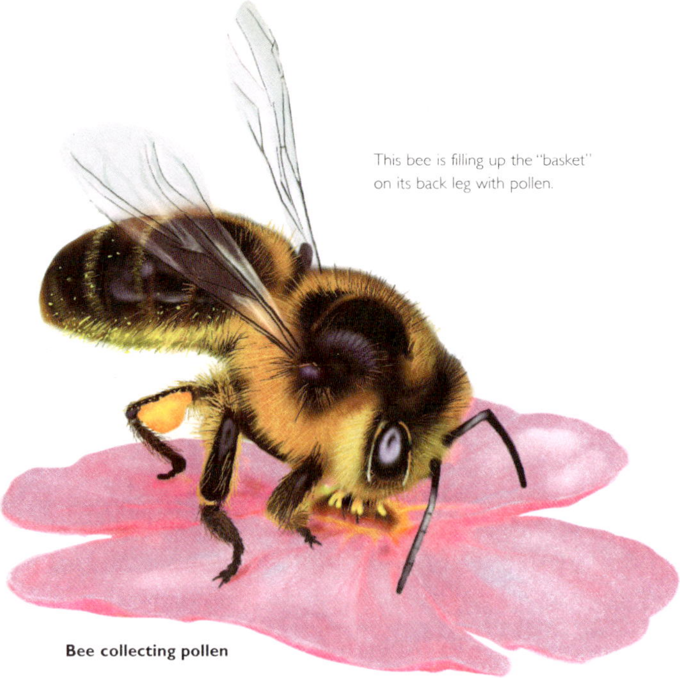

This bee is filling up the "basket" on its back leg with pollen.

**Bee collecting pollen**

# How many bees live in a hive?

IN A BUSY HIVE THERE CAN BE UP TO 80,000 HONEYBEE WORKERS.

There will be just one adult queen bee. She may live for as long as five years, and she is the most important member of the hive. The worker bees have an adult life of only about 6 weeks. The hive may also contain up to 200 male bees (drones) whose only job is to fertilize the queen on a mating flight. Bumblebees have much smaller nests than honeybees. The nest only lasts one season.

### Are bees vegetarian?

Yes, bees, unlike their relatives the wasps, are vegetarian. They feed on nectar from flowers. Honeybees have tongues that are made for sucking nectar from shallow flowers. Many bumblebees have longer tongues that can push deep into tube-shaped flowers. Bees also collect pollen from flowers, to take back to the nest to fed their young.

### What is bee-bread?

Bee-bread is the mixture of honey and pollen that bees use as food, particularly to feed the larvae that will grow up to be workers.

### How do bees become queens?

The job that a bee does in the hive depends on what it eats. A queen bee has a special diet. The workers build some large cells for the young queens, and start special treatment for them. They are fed on rich food, called royal jelly, produced by glands in the workers' heads. This allows them to develop into full queens. Only some bees are queens, because the adult queen in a hive makes a chemical that spreads round all the workers and stops them from becoming queens. If the queen gets weak, or the hive is very large, there is not enough of this chemical to work and it no longer has an effect.

### How many flowers a day does a bee visit?

A honeybee makes about 10 trips from the hive, each day, looking for food. It can take up to 1,000 flowers to provide enough nectar for a bee on a trip. So, it could be visiting around 10,000 flowers a day.

**A bee's waggle dance**

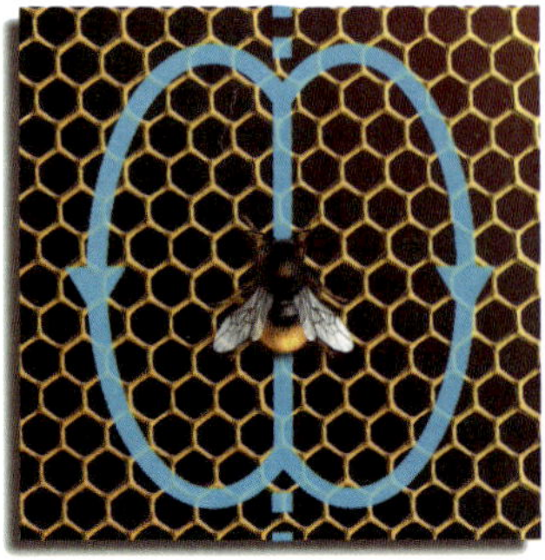

### Why are bees good dancers?

When a bee returns from a successful trip to find pollen, it "dances" on the top of the honeycomb, surrounded by other workers. Its movements during the dance tell the other bees how far away the food source is, and the angle to the sun at which they must fly to reach it.

**How long have people kept bees?**
People have made use of bees for a very long time. Beehives, and their keepers, are shown in ancient Egyptian paintings from 5,000 years ago.

**Why are bees hairy?**
Some bumblebees are quite good at keeping themselves warm, when the outside temperature is low, and their furry bodies probably help with this. For most bees, though, a hairy body is useful mainly because it gathers up pollen grains, from the flowers as it looks for nectar.

**Where is a bee's shopping basket?**
Many bees have a special brush of hairs on each back leg, that they use as a shopping basket. When they have collected pollen on their body hairs, they clean it off, and gather it all into the pollen basket on the leg. You can often spot a well-filled, yellow pollen basket on a bee.

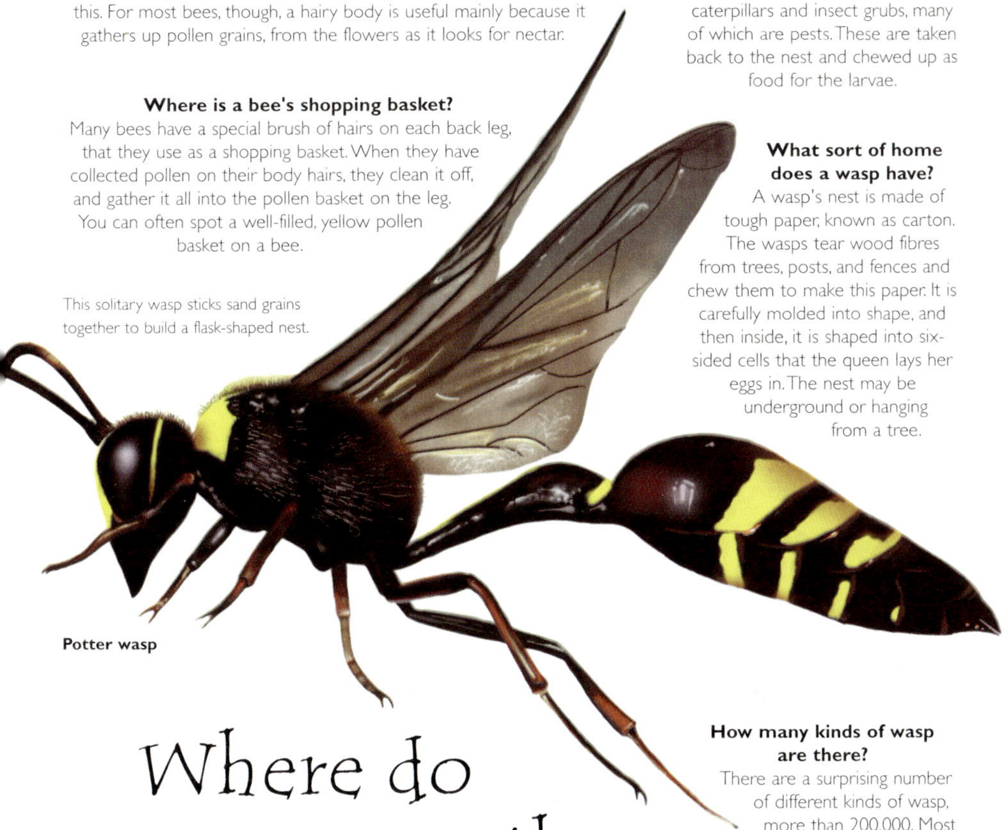

This solitary wasp sticks sand grains together to build a flask-shaped nest.

**Potter wasp**

# Where do wasps go in the winter?

UNLIKE HONEYBEES, WASPS DO NOT STORE UP SWEET SUBSTANCES IN THEIR NESTS, so the colony has nothing to survive on in the winter. At the end of the summer, after the new queens have mated, the workers all die. Just the queen survives the winter in hibernation, and she starts a new colony in the spring.

**Are wasps any use?**
Many people think that the yellow and black striped wasps are our enemies. These wasps do have a powerful sting, but it is not often used against humans. In fact, they do an enormous amount of good for people, as they collect a lot of caterpillars and insect grubs, many of which are pests. These are taken back to the nest and chewed up as food for the larvae.

**What sort of home does a wasp have?**
A wasp's nest is made of tough paper, known as carton. The wasps tear wood fibres from trees, posts, and fences and chew them to make this paper. It is carefully molded into shape, and then inside, it is shaped into six-sided cells that the queen lays her eggs in. The nest may be underground or hanging from a tree.

**How many kinds of wasp are there?**
There are a surprising number of different kinds of wasp, more than 200,000. Most of them are not the familiar striped social wasps, but are types such as sawflies, wood wasps, sand wasps, and other kinds of hunting wasp.

**Which wasp eats its victims alive?**
There are lots of parasitic wasps. These wasps paralyze their victim then lay their eggs inside its body. When the eggs hatch, the larvae feed on the victim from inside it, while it is still alive.

### Does the female mantis eat her mate?

In some species of mantis the male is at risk of being the female's dinner, if he does not avoid her clutches. The first part to be eaten is usually the male's head. Unbelievably, this does not stop it mating.

### What is the mantis's main weapon?

The front legs of the mantis are its main weapons. They are very spiny and great for seizing their prey, rather like spiny pincers. They are also good as a defence against attackers. Even humans can get a nasty jab from a mantis if it swivels its front legs and uses its spines to stab.

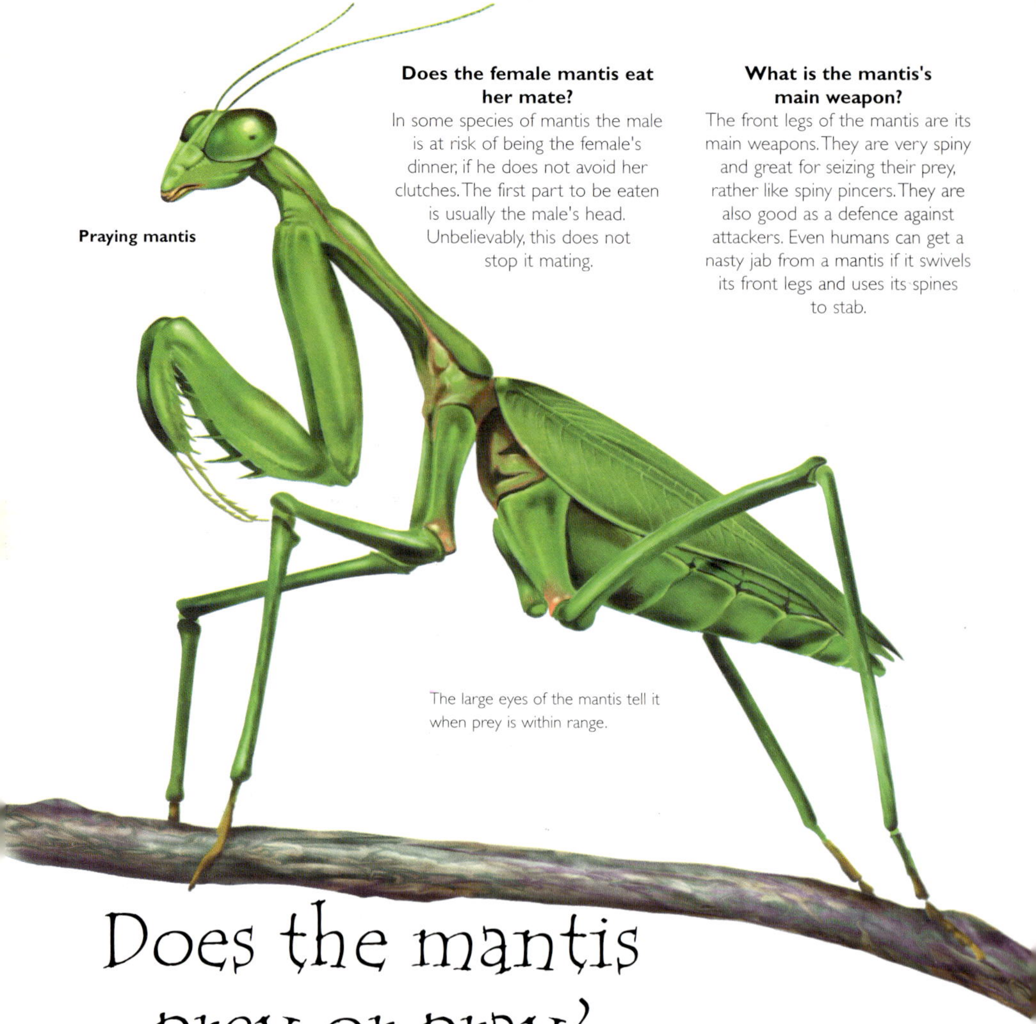

**Praying mantis**

The large eyes of the mantis tell it when prey is within range.

# Does the mantis prey or pray?

THE MANTIS OF THE MEDITERRANEAN AREA IS CALLED THE "PRAYING mantis" because of the way that it sits, with its front legs folded up in front of its head, as if it was saying its prayers. It does its share of preying as well. It is a fierce carnivore that will grab and eat insects and even small animals.

### How long is the longest stick insect?

The longest stick insect is the saw-footed stick insect of South-east Asia. It grows up to 13 in (33 cm) long – as long as a pet rabbit.

### Why are male stick insects rare?

In many, but not all, species of stick insects males are just not needed. Some species, such as the "laboratory" stick insect, manage perfectly well with no males at all. The females can produce eggs without mating, and these develop into more females, just like their parent.

### Can a praying mantis fly?

Many mantis females have small, useless wings, or no wings at all. Adult male mantises, though, have fully developed wings and may fly off if attacked.

**How does a stick insect disguise its eggs?**

A stick insect lays eggs that look like seeds. They are dropped on the ground, and scattered one by one. They have a hard shell with a cap at one end, through which the young will eventually hatch. This may take up to three years, so its very important that they look like a tough seed, rather than a tasty morsel.

**What do adult dragonflies eat?**

Adult dragonflies catch other insects in mid-air. They hold all their spiny legs out forwards to make a catching basket. Into this fly flies, beetles, and even bees, where they are bitten by the powerful jaws of the dragonfly. Sometimes dragonflies scoop up their prey from plants or from the ground.

**Why does a dragonfly need a mask?**

A dragonfly larva needs a mask in order to eat. The mask is the lower jaw that can be pushed outward. When the dragonfly is resting, the jaw covers a lot of the face, just like a mask. The larva lives in water and preys on insects, small fish, and tadpoles. The mask is hinged, and can be shot out suddenly. Two hooks on the end stab the prey, so it can be pulled back into the mouth.

# What is the biggest dragonfly?

THE LARGEST DRAGONFLIES OF THE PRESENT DAY ARE SOUTH American giant damselflies. They have a wingspan of up to 7 in (19 cm), with a body 5 in (12 cm) long. These are dwarfs, though, compared with dragonflies that lived 280 million years ago. Fossils have been found with a wingspan of 29 in (75 cm). That means they would have been about the size of a small dog.

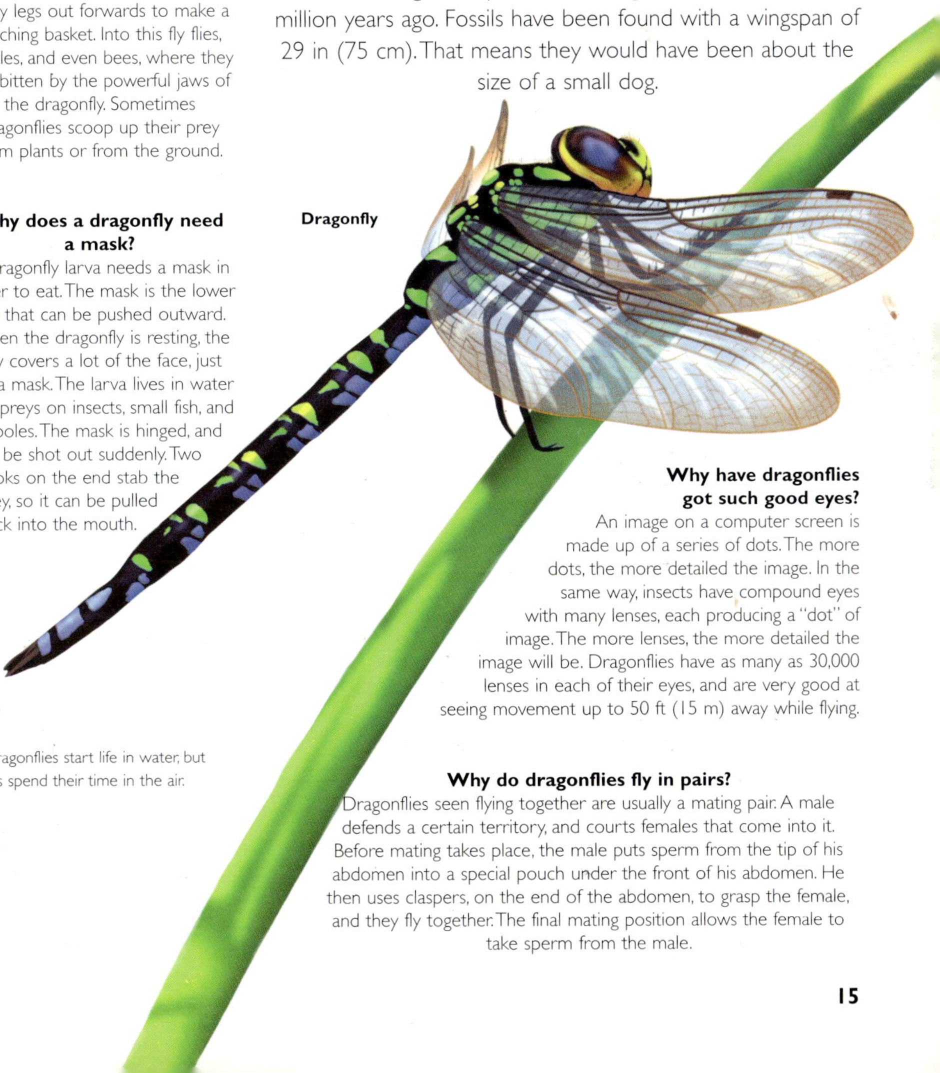

Dragonfly

All dragonflies start life in water, but adults spend their time in the air.

**Why have dragonflies got such good eyes?**

An image on a computer screen is made up of a series of dots. The more dots, the more detailed the image. In the same way, insects have compound eyes with many lenses, each producing a "dot" of image. The more lenses, the more detailed the image will be. Dragonflies have as many as 30,000 lenses in each of their eyes, and are very good at seeing movement up to 50 ft (15 m) away while flying.

**Why do dragonflies fly in pairs?**

Dragonflies seen flying together are usually a mating pair. A male defends a certain territory, and courts females that come into it. Before mating takes place, the male puts sperm from the tip of his abdomen into a special pouch under the front of his abdomen. He then uses claspers, on the end of the abdomen, to grasp the female, and they fly together. The final mating position allows the female to take sperm from the male.

# How do cicadas sing?

ANYONE WHO HAS BEEN IN A WARM COUNTRY HAS HEARD THE LOUD calls of cicadas. These bugs make their sound using a kind of drumskin on each side of their abdomen. This skin is pulled in by a muscle, then allowed to snap out again, producing one click in the group of clicks that make up the cicada's song. Air sacs help to increase the sound.

**Which bugs feed on human blood?**
A number of assassin bugs can feed on human blood, but most are not dangerous. One, however is dangerous, not because of the blood it takes, but because it carries a disease. The South American bug *Triatoma infestans* carries the germ that causes Chagas' disease. This illness gives a high fever and a swollen liver, spleen, and lymph nodes.

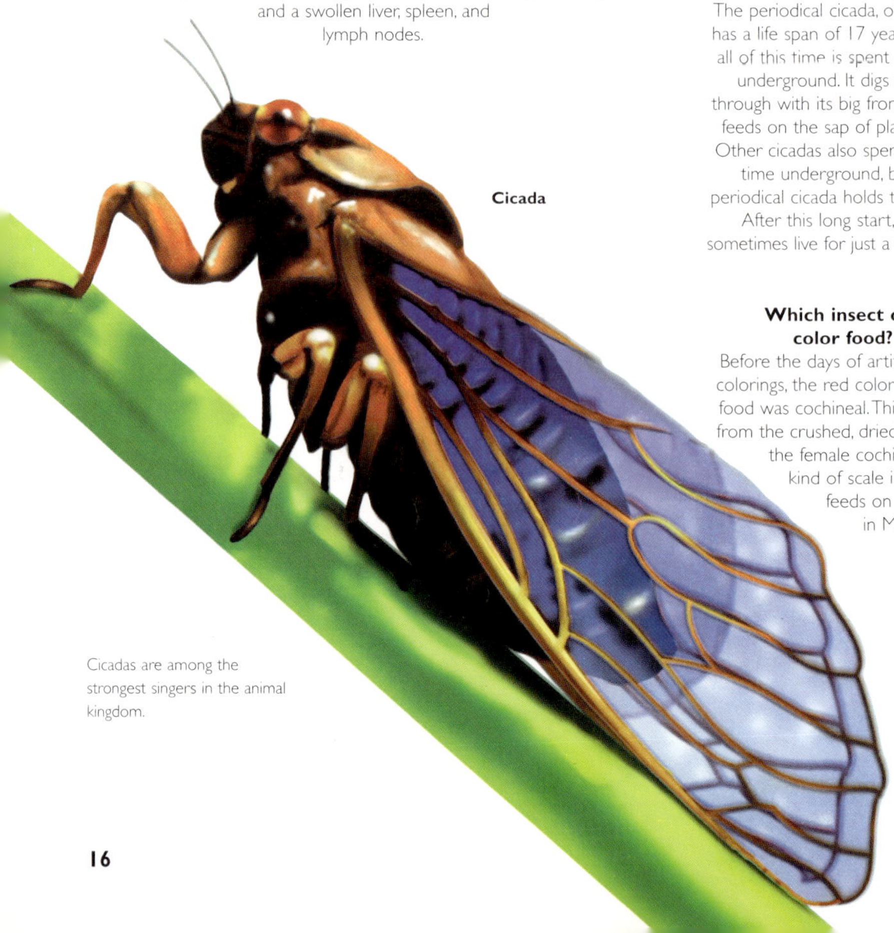

Cicada

Cicadas are among the strongest singers in the animal kingdom.

**Which bug is an assassin?**
Assassin bugs are predators (creatures that prey on other creatures) that use their piercing, sucking mouthparts to impale insects, so that they can feed on their body fluids. They inject digestive juices and suck up the resulting "soup." They may carry their prey on their beaks. A few species suck the blood of animals.

**What insect makes sweets?**
Some kinds of scaled insects produce a syrupy secretion. As the insect produces the secretion, it dries quickly in the hot climate to form sugary, honeydew lumps. It can then be eaten by humans.

**Which bug spends years underground?**
The periodical cicada, of America, has a life span of 17 years. Almost all of this time is spent as a larva underground. It digs its way through with its big front legs, and feeds on the sap of plant roots. Other cicadas also spend a lot of time underground, but the periodical cicada holds the record. After this long start, adults sometimes live for just a few weeks.

**Which insect can color food?**
Before the days of artificial food colorings, the red color added to food was cochineal. This is made from the crushed, dried bodies of the female cochineal bug, a kind of scale insect that feeds on cacti in Mexico.

**What is cuckoo-spit?**
Cuckoo-spit does not come from cuckoos. The frothy "spit" is made by a frog hopper larva. It blows air into a liquid that comes from its anus. The froth that it produces protects the larva from enemies, as well as keeping it moist. Adult frog hopper bugs are very good at hopping, which is why they are called hopper bugs.

**How do aphids drink plant juice?**
Aphids, such as the greenfly that you find on roses, have special piercing tools on their mouths that point downwards. These are pushed down into the plant vein, and act just like a straw. They inject saliva down one channel of the mouthparts and suck up juices through another.

**How do aphids cause havoc?**
Sometimes aphids damage crops just because there are so many of them sucking sap, and weakening or killing the plants. In other cases the plants develop deformed leaves that make them useless to sell. Those aphids that fly from plant to plant can also spread serious diseases, injecting them into the plant as they suck sap.

**Which insect doesn't like wine?**
The vine phylloxera aphid comes from North America. It was accidentally introduced to Europe in the 19th century, where it destroyed thousands of the grape vines.

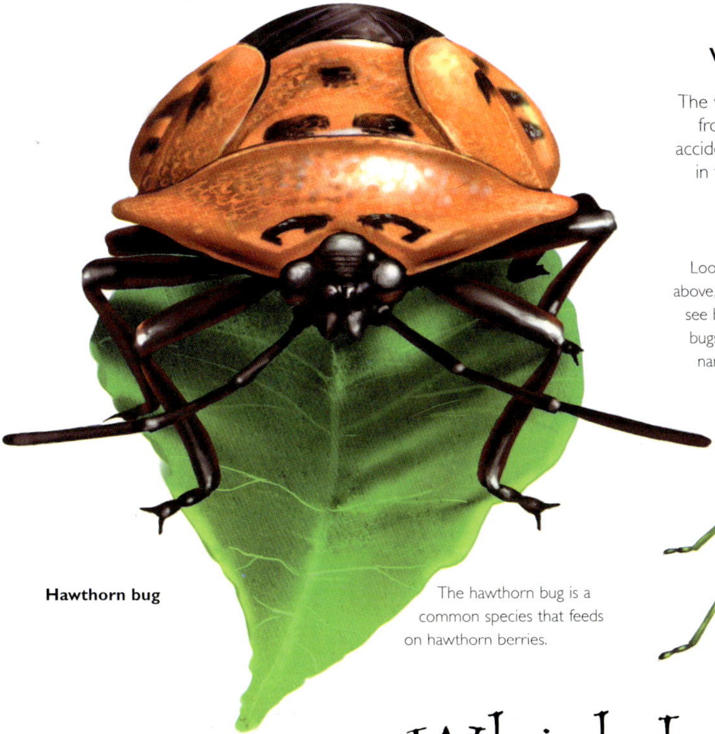

**Hawthorn bug**

The hawthorn bug is a common species that feeds on hawthorn berries.

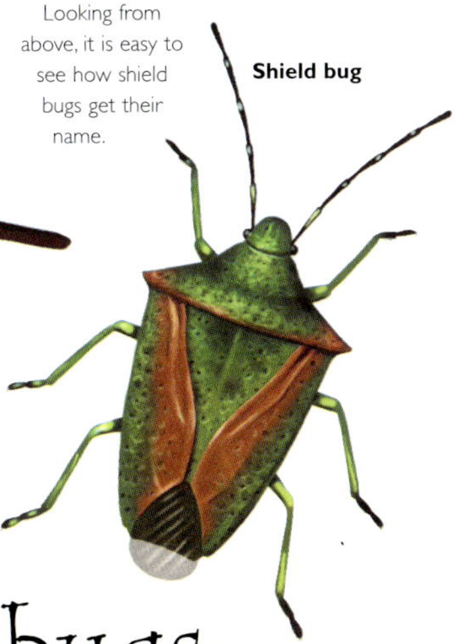

Looking from above, it is easy to see how shield bugs get their name.

**Shield bug**

# Which bugs stink?

THE SHIELD BUG HAS QUITE A FLAT BODY, THAT LOOKS LIKE A SHIELD WHEN seen from above. It lives on plants, which they eat with their piercing mouthparts. They have glands in their body which produce a smell. In some cases this smells really strong to humans, which is how this bug earned the name stink bug.

**Which bug followed us from our ancestors' caves?**
The bed-bug is a wingless insect that comes out at night, and feeds on human blood. In the day, it hides in small, dark places. Bed-bugs attack other warm-blooded animals too. They probably first started attacking humans when our ancestors lived in caves close to other animals. Piles of skins and fur would have provided ideal hideaways. Bed-bugs are rarely a problem in hygienic modern houses.

**How do some grasshoppers disappear in a flash?**
Most grasshoppers are brown or green in color, and patterned for camouflage. But many have hind wings that are a bright contrasting color. This is "flash coloration." If an enemy comes too close, the grasshopper suddenly takes flight, showing the bright hind wings. This can startle and put off a predator. Alternatively, if the predator watches the bright wings, it can be confused when the insect suddenly lands, and disappears behind its camouflage.

**Which crickets like to make a noise?**
The mole cricket spends much of its time burrowing underground. On summer nights, it makes a burrow that is just the right shape to increase the noises it makes. (This is the same shape that humans have come up with to make their stereo amplifiers!). The cricket sits in the entrance singing continuously. The amplifier is so successful that the cricket can be heard a mile away.

**Do grasshoppers have ears?**
Yes, but they aren't always where you'd expect them to be. Short-horned grasshoppers do not have ears on their heads, but on their abdomens. In crickets and their relatives, they are on their legs. Each ear has a thin "eardrum" which vibrates when sounds hit it.

Good eyesight and hearing warn a grasshopper of approaching enemies.

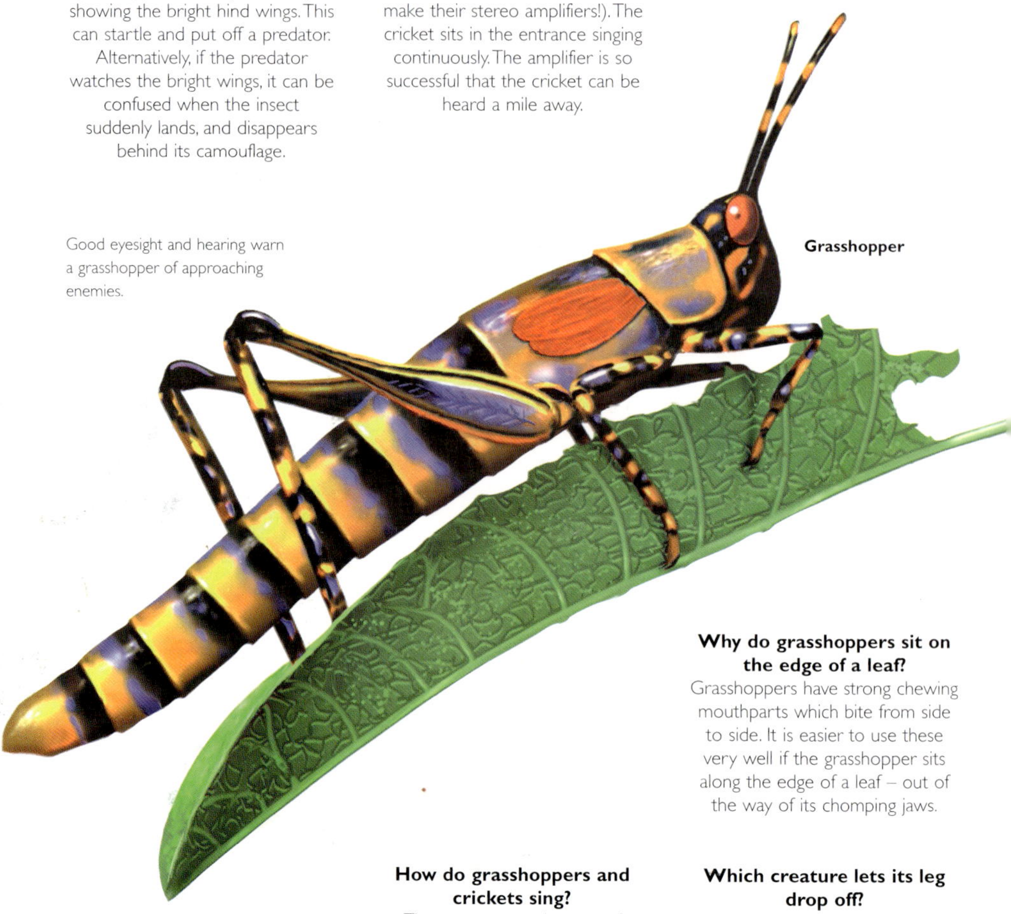

Grasshopper

**Why do grasshoppers sit on the edge of a leaf?**
Grasshoppers have strong chewing mouthparts which bite from side to side. It is easier to use these very well if the grasshopper sits along the edge of a leaf – out of the way of its chomping jaws.

**Why are crickets kept in cages?**
In China, the song of the house cricket has always been really popular, even in the emperor's court. So, there is a Chinese tradition of keeping crickets in small cages to hear their song. Only the male cricket sings. He may chirp 10,000 times an hour.

**How do grasshoppers and crickets sing?**
There are two main ways of "singing" if you are a grasshopper or cricket. Short-horned grasshoppers scratch a row of projections (something that sticks up) from the inside of the hind leg against the veins of the front wing. In other grasshoppers and crickets, the bases of the front wings are scratched together to make the sound.

**Which creature lets its leg drop off?**
If another animal seizes a grasshopper by the leg, the grasshopper will throw its own leg off, rather than let itself be caught. A special lining quickly seals the hole, so that the grasshopper doesn't lose much blood. A grasshopper can work surprisingly well with only one of its long jumping legs to work with.

# What is a locust?

LOCUSTS ARE SPECIES OF GRASSHOPPER. THE UNUSUAL THING ABOUT them is that at times they form huge swarms. Most locusts live alone, just like the average grasshopper, but when conditions are right, and there is plenty of food around, they join together to form massive swarms.

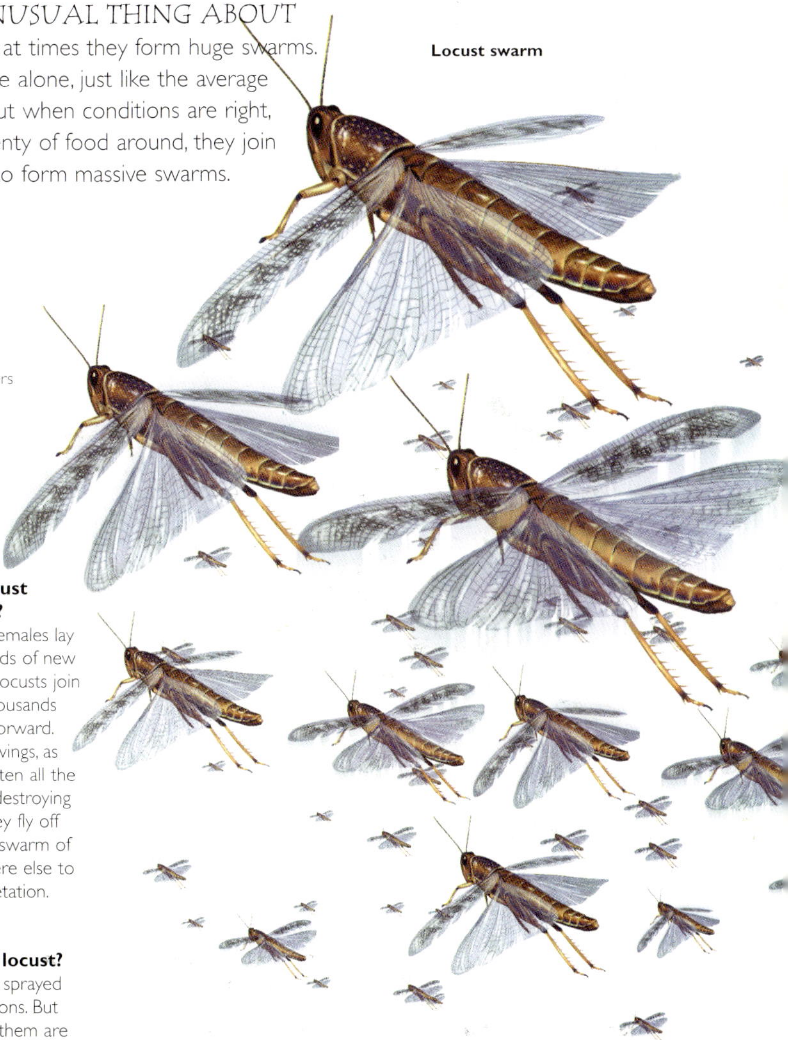

Locust swarm

Each locust has a moderate appetite, but the vast numbers in a swarm can cause devastation to crops.

**How does a locust swarm form?**
When the rains come, females lay lots of eggs and thousands of new locusts are born. All the locusts join together, and soon thousands of them are moving forward. By the time they get wings, as adults, they may have eaten all the food in the area. After destroying all the crops there, they fly off again and the terrifying swarm of locusts arrives somewhere else to strip the land of vegetation.

**How do you stop a locust?**
Locust swarms can be sprayed from the air with poisons. But by the time millions of them are flying together, they are difficult to stop. Nowadays, scientists keep an eye on locust numbers, to make sure they aren't building up too much. If they see a dramatic increase in locust numbers, they can often be destroyed before they get out of control.

**Where do locusts live?**
Locusts live in the Mediterranean region, Asia, Australia, North and South America. The most destructive of all are the migratory locust, and the desert locust, which live in Africa and the Middle East and can destroy crops in just a few minutes.

**How many locusts are there in a swarm?**
Many millions of locusts move together in the largest swarms. The biggest may cover hundreds of square miles and contain 50,000 million locusts. A swarm like that would weigh as much as 50,000 people.

# How high can a flea jump?

HUMAN FLEAS CAN JUMP UP TO 7 IN (20 CM) HIGH, AND CAT FLEAS EVEN higher, up to 13 in (34 cm). This is an amazing jump when you think that fleas are so tiny. Fleas can store energy in a membrane of elastic protein, and it is when this is released that they are clicked into the air.

**What do young fleas look like?**
Young fleas are tiny, worm-like larvae. The larva lives in the nest on the animal its living on, and feeds on drops of dry blood from the faeces of the adults. After two or three weeks, it turns into a pupa (the stage just before it becomes an adult). It may wait some time before hatching out. The movement of the host animal stirs the adult fleas into moving.

**How big do fleas get?**
The size of the host makes no difference to the size of the flea that attacks it. The biggest flea in Britain is the mole flea, about ¼ in (6 mm) long (the size of a small fly). The world record is held by an American flea. It was a flea from a mountain beaver, and it was ⅓ in (8 mm) long.

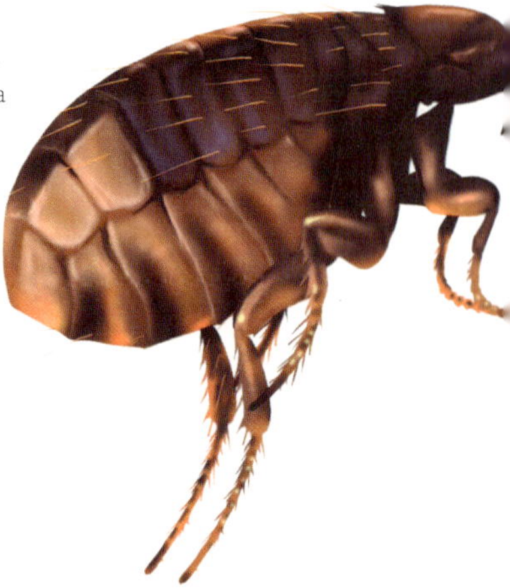

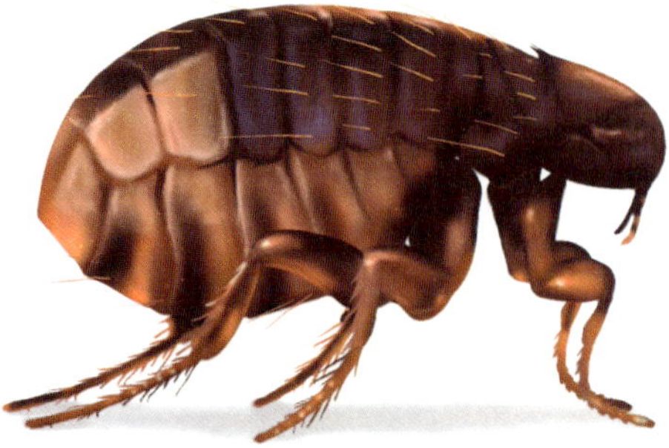

Fleas

It is elastic under tension, rather than muscle effort, that powers the flea's jump.

**Do birds have fleas?**
Nine-tenths of the world's fleas feed on mammals, but there are species that attack birds. Because fleas don't have wings they cannot move very far, so they need to live somewhere where they can find lots of hosts to live on. They tend to live in bird nests.

**Why do fleas spread the plague?**
Plague is a disease that is carried by rats. Fleas that carry the disease live on rats and can then jump onto humans and bite them. The plague spreads very quickly. Outbreaks in the Middle Ages, such as the Black Death, wiped out half the human population in some areas of Europe. Outbreaks of plague still occur.

**Do fleas like to live on anyone?**
Fleas do tend to live on just one particular type of host. There are cat fleas and dog fleas, for example, that live in the fur of these animals. Rabbits, porcupines, and beavers have their own fleas. "Human" fleas on the other hand, are shared with foxes and pigs. If they are hungry enough, most fleas will take blood from any animal. Human fleas are now rare in houses, and genuine dog fleas are not very common in Britain. Most fleas around now are cat fleas.

**What are nits?**
Nits are the eggs of the head louse. Female lice lay eggs in the hair of the human host. They stick to the hair of the host because if they fell off they would die. A fine comb is often used to remove nits from hair.

**Why do lice have flat bodies?**
Lice have low, flat bodies so that they can squeeze between the hairs of the host. They also have short legs that allow them to hold tight if the host tries to scratch them off. Fleas are flat for the same reasons.

**What are jiggers?**
Jiggers are also called sand fleas. The females burrow into the skin of animals, including the feet of humans. Here they remain for the rest of their lives, laying the eggs that will produce the next generation.

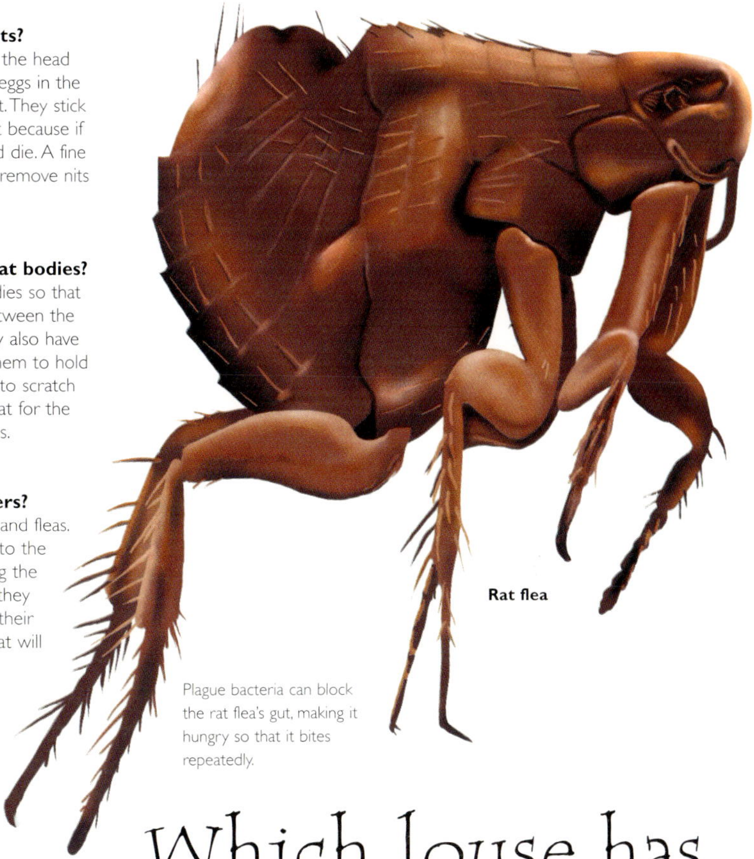

**Rat flea**

Plague bacteria can block the rat flea's gut, making it hungry so that it bites repeatedly.

**What do lice eat?**
All lice are parasites. They live on the skin of mammals and birds. One group has chewing mouthparts, and feeds on flakes of skin, feather, sweat, or blood. Another group of lice has piercing and sucking mouthparts and feeds on mammal's blood. Human lice belong to this group.

**Are head lice dangerous?**
The human head louse lives in human hair and can be an irritating nuisance. But it is not dangerous and doesn't spread disease. It will live on clean hair as happily as dirty. Lice cannot fly, so they like to live in crowded conditions where they can easily step from one human head to another, to get a new feeding ground.

# Which louse has killed millions of people?

THE HUMAN BODY LOUSE HAS BEEN RESPONSIBLE FOR KILLING VAST numbers of people. When people are crowded in dirty conditions, in wars or natural disasters, body lice can thrive and multiply. Unfortunately, they can carry typhus. This disease is a killer. It is thought to have caused the deaths of some 3,000,000 people in Eastern Europe in the First World War (1914–18), and to have killed more people in concentration camps in the Second World War (1939–45) than any other cause.

# How do flies feed?

THE FLY LANDS ON THE FOOD – A PIECE OF MEAT OR CHEESE – AND SPITS ON IT TO soften it. All flies have sucking mouthparts, with pumping muscles in the head, and it uses these to suck up the softened food. In many flies, the tip of the mouthparts spreads out to form a sponge to absorb the liquid food. Some, such as horse-flies and mosquitoes, have piercing mouthparts, and take blood from whatever they are feeding on.

**Why are fruit-flies important to scientists?**
Fruit-flies are important because they are small and easily bred in captivity, and have a speedy life history. Scientists have been able to use them to find out an enormous amount about how genes (the units that pass from generation to generation and make us the same as our parents) work.

**Why do some flies look like bees?**
By trying to look like animals with a dangerous sting, flies may stop many animals from attacking them. The hoverflies, in particular, look like and behave like bees and wasps. The hoverfly *Volucella bombylans* actually has different forms mimicking different bumblebees. It lays eggs in bumblebee nests too, where its larvae steal the food meant for the bumblebee larvae.

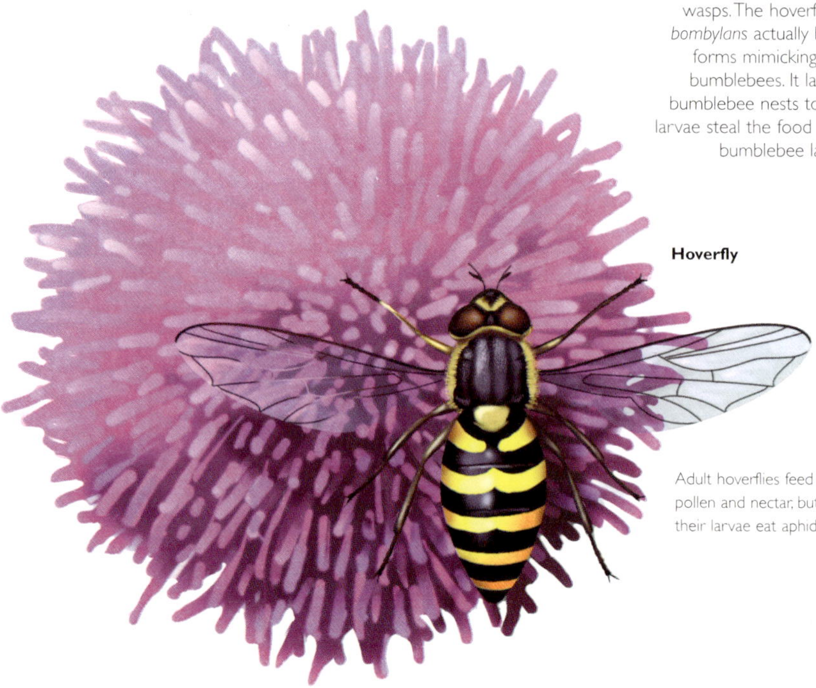

**Hoverfly**

Adult hoverflies feed on pollen and nectar, but their larvae eat aphids.

**Why do flies like animal dung?**
Many species of fly lay their eggs on dung, which provides a nourishing food for the larva. The true dung flies have legless larvae which wriggle their way about, sucking in food greedily, until they have grown enough to turn into pupae in the soil below a cow-pat.

**Can flies eat your living flesh?**
Some flies lay their eggs in the skin of living animals. The larvae hatch and burrow into flesh and feed on it. The warble flies eat the flesh of cattle and deer, causing much irritation. The tumbu fly larva, of Africa, lives under the skin of humans.

**How do bluebottles spread disease?**
Bluebottles eat the kind of food that is likely to have bacteria on it, such as rotting vegetation or faeces. Often, they will then land on our food, carrying the disease with them to infect an unfortunate human with diarrhoea, or worse.

**Can you tell a fly by its wings?**
True flies can always be recognised among the insects because they have a single pair of wings rather than four. In fact, the rear wings have been turned into stabilizers. They are club-shaped projections (areas that stick out) from the body that give the fly information about how it is flying.

**Why do humans avoid the tsetse fly?**
The tsetse fly is the insect that carries sleeping sickness, and can give it to humans. The disease is quite common in wild grazing animals, and doesn't affect them badly, but it can be devastating to humans. Because it is such a serious disease, humans try to live in areas where the tsetse fly is not known to live.

**Which flies help the police with their enquiries?**
Different species of flies arrive at different stages, during the rotting of flesh, to lay their eggs. The larvae grow, pupate, and then turn into adults to a fast timetable. This allows a forensic scientist (scientists who study how people have died) to make a good estimate of the time of death. They look at what flies, at what stage of growth, are in a dead body.

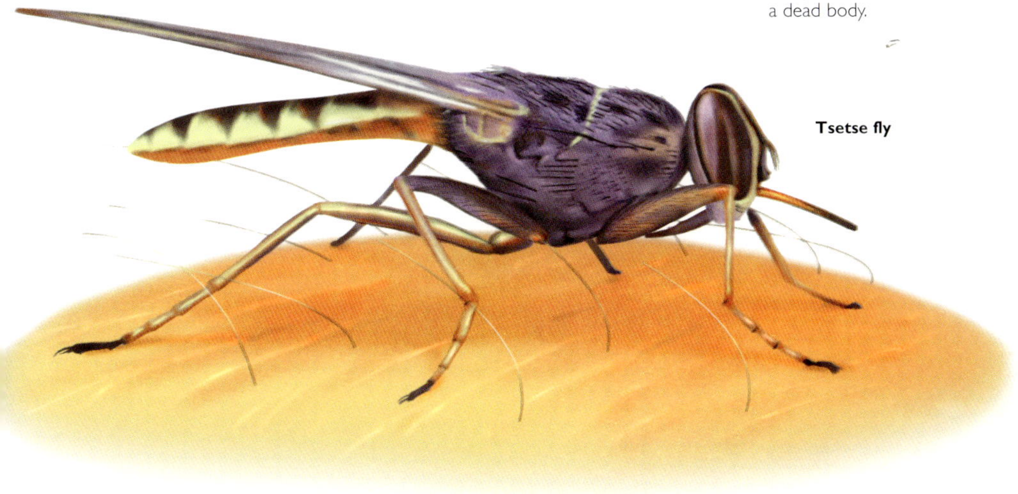


The tsetse fly carries the parasite that causes sleeping sickness.

# Why are mosquitoes our deadly enemies?

THE FEMALE MOSQUITO IS A BLOODSUCKER, BUT THE DISEASES SHE MAY CARRY IN her saliva are the real danger to humans. In the warmer parts of the world, there is always a danger that a mosquito is carrying the germ that causes malaria. This disease affects a large section of the world population and it makes people very weak and ill.

**How does a blowfly taste its food?**
It is useful to a fly to know, before it tries to feed, whether what it has landed on is a possible food. The fly has special tasters, in the hairs on its feet, that tell it whether it's on food or not. These hairs may be much more sensitive than the human tongue.

**What are "no-see-ums'?**
No-see-ums are North American biting midges. They feed on us, using piercing mouthparts to take blood. Biting midges are all very small flies, but those that attack humans have an irritating bite. Being so small, they often manage to bite before being noticed, which is where the name comes from.

Longhorn beetles, like this *Strangalia,* are often striking looking. They live in the open as adults. But, their larval life is usually spent boring into wood.

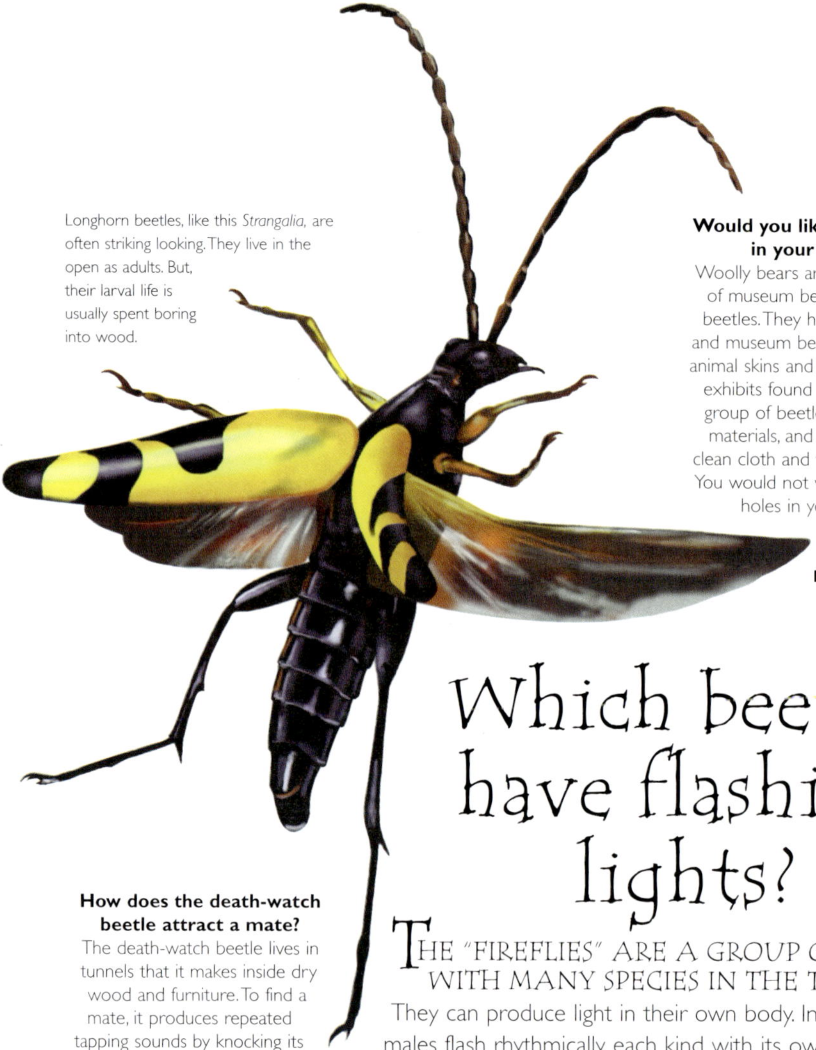

**Longhorn beetle**

### Would you like a woolly bear in your sweater?

Woolly bears are the hairy larvae of museum beetles and carpet beetles. They have a varied diet, and museum beetles will eat dried animal skins and many of the other exhibits found in museums. This group of beetles is also fond of materials, and particularly fine, clean cloth and woollen garments. You would not want one gnawing holes in your sweater.

# Which beetles have flashing lights?

THE "FIREFLIES" ARE A GROUP OF BEETLES WITH MANY SPECIES IN THE TROPICS. They can produce light in their own body. In many species males flash rhythmically, each kind with its own code. In the glow-worm, of Europe, the wingless female gives off a greenish light from her body to attract the males.

### How does the death-watch beetle attract a mate?

The death-watch beetle lives in tunnels that it makes inside dry wood and furniture. To find a mate, it produces repeated tapping sounds by knocking its head on the floor of the tunnel. The sounds are rather like a ticking clock.

### Which beetle might you find in your cereal?

A number of beetles can get into cereal products such as flour, grain, and biscuits. Apart from weevils there are the large mealworm beetle and the flour beetle. They get into stores in warehouses, and their larvae damage everything that they touch. Flour beetles can infest houses too and eat all the dry food in your cupboards.

### Which is the largest beetle?

The biggest beetles in the world are about the size of a mouse. Several tropical beetles are this size, including the rhinoceros beetle of South America. The heaviest beetle measured was a goliath beetle from Africa, weighing in at 3½ oz (100 g).

### Why do ladybirds have bright colors?

Many beetles that are brightly colored in red or yellow, like the ladybird, are telling predators that they aren't very nice to eat. Ladybirds will also bleed from their leg joints when attacked, letting out sticky, toxic blood which repels and gums up an attacker.

# Why were dung beetles sacred?

THE SCARAB DUNG BEETLES WERE SACRED IN ANCIENT EGYPT BECAUSE THE Egyptians thought they were linked to the gods they worshipped. These beetles gather a ball of dung that they roll away to a hole, as food for their young. To the ancient Egyptians this ball symbolized the globe of the sun, being pushed across the sky each day by the sun god.

**How many beetle species are there?**
About 370,000 different species of beetles have been found so far; that's one third of all the known animals in the world. Beetle specialists can only guess how many more await discovery, particularly in the tropics. Estimates suggest that at least as many again will be found, and there could be up to 5,000,000 species. Beetles are easily the biggest group of animals in the world.

**Which beetles shoot their enemies?**
Bombardier beetles store chemicals in a special chamber in their body. If they are attacked, the chemicals react to produce a boiling hot mixture that can blister skin. These are shot, like explosives, from a nozzle in the body. They are so hot that they become an irritating gas cloud that repels an attacker.

**How are dung beetles useful?**
Dung beetles remove and break down vast amounts of dung, and return its goodness to the soil. In Australia there were no insects to deal with the dung produced by cattle, so dung beetles were imported from Africa to help to solve this problem.

**Is a weevil evil?**
The weevils are a huge group of beetles, that have "elbows" on their antennae. Many weevils are a minor nuisance. Some species are major pests, like the boll weevil that lives inside cotton flowers, and stops cotton fibres from growing. Other species cause serious damage in stored grain.

**Dung beetle**

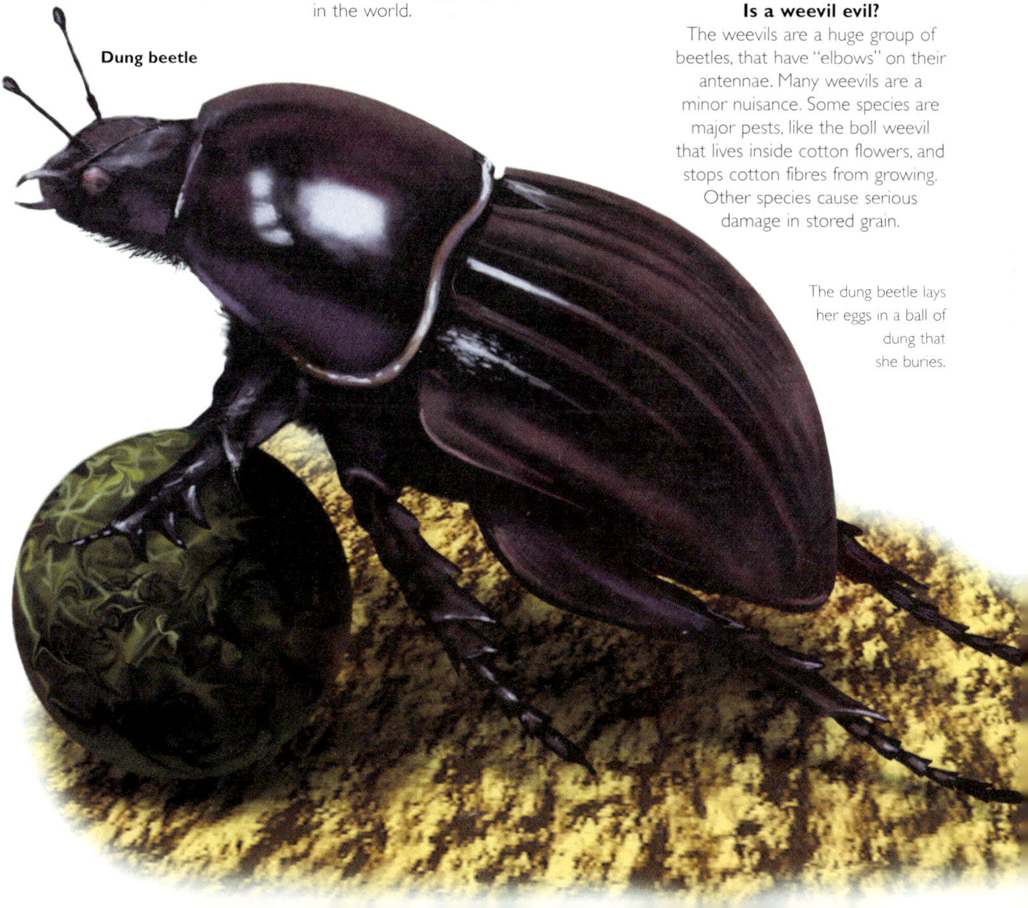

The dung beetle lays her eggs in a ball of dung that she buries.

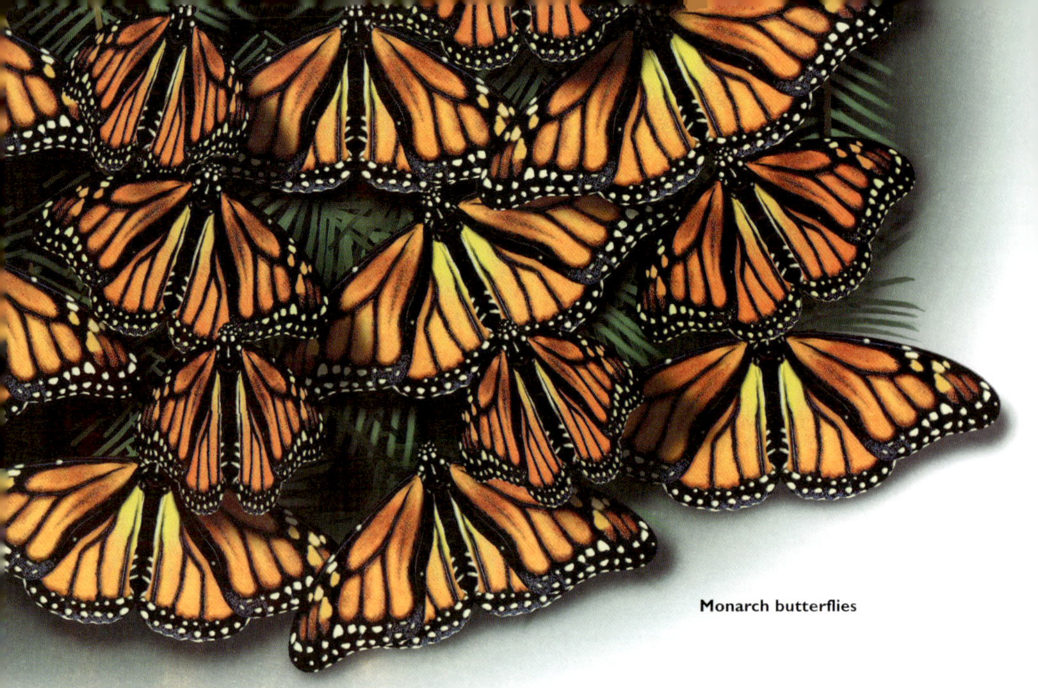

Monarch butterflies

In winter, monarch butterflies roost together in vast numbers.

# How far can butterflies fly?

MANY BUTTERFLIES FLY VERY WELL. RED ADMIRAL AND PAINTED LADY butterflies do not normally survive the winter in Britain. Some North American monarch butterflies fly to Mexico, to spend the winter in huge communal roosts. They can fly 1,180 miles (1,900 km) in just three weeks.

**How do you tell a butterfly from a moth?**

Butterflies fly by day, have club-shaped antennae, and are often brightly colored. Moths fly by night, have feathery antennae, and are duller in color.

**What do butterflies like to eat?**

Adult butterflies do not need to grow, so their food needs are for energy, rather than protein. The typical butterfly food is nectar from flowers. However, some feed on sap oozing from trees, from rotting fruit, and some, including some of the most beautiful, from dung. They will also take in salts from mud.

**Where do butterflies go in the winter?**

In cooler climates, when butterflies disappear in winter, many people assume they all die. Some do, but some species spend the winter hibernating before breeding the next year. In Britain, these include brimstone, peacock, and small tortoiseshell butterflies. In other parts of the world, butterflies may migrate with the seasons. The North American monarch butterfly spends its winter in sunny Mexico.

**How are the colors of butterflies made?**

The wings of butterflies and moths are covered in tiny overlapping scales (their scientific name, *Lepidoptera,* means scaled wings). Each individual scale can be filled with color, giving the insect its characteristic pattern. In some butterflies, such as the shiny tropical *Morpho* butterflies, the color is produced by the special structure of the scale as much as the color on it.

# Are moths poisonous?

MOTHS DO NOT HAVE A POISONOUS BITE, BUT MANY ARE POISONOUS TO animals that bite them. Often their colors advertize that they have chemical defences. The cinnabar moth has a caterpillar, with black and yellow warning colors, that feeds on ragwort, a plant with poisonous sap. The caterpillar isn't affected by the poison and stores it in its own body. For the rest of its life it carries the poison which only affects those that attack it, never the moth itself.

The eyespots of the emperor moth make it look like the face of a bigger animal.

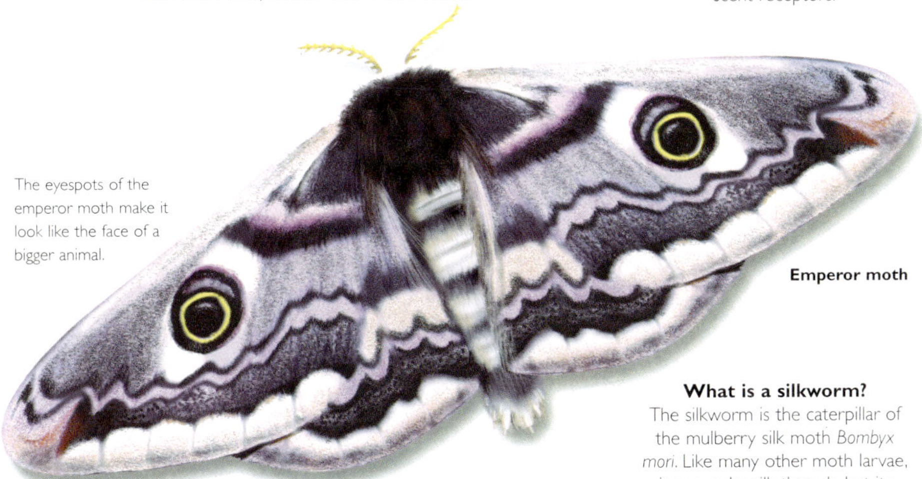

**Emperor moth**

**Which moth encourages its food to grow?**

Many moths and butterflies may help their food grow, because they help to pollinate flowers. The yucca moths of Mexico and North America lay their eggs in the ovaries of the yucca flower, then put pollen on the stigma so the flower is fertilized. By doing this it is helping the plant to produce seeds. Of the seeds it produces, some may grow into new plants, but many will be eaten by the moth larvae that are developing within the ovary. Both the moth and the plant benefit.

**Why do butterflies and moths have eyespots?**

The eyespots on the wings of a moth or butterfly can fool a predator into thinking it is a larger animal, and therefore leaves it alone. If it is attacked, the eyespots are more noticeable than the body and head. This can be a lifesaver, if a bird goes for these first, it leaves the butterfly in one piece, apart from a slice out of the wing.

**How do tiger moths baffle bats?**

Bats hunt tiger moths at night. The bats give out high-pitched sounds, and find their prey from the echo that the sounds produce. Tiger moths have "eardrums" on their body. They hear the bats' cries and keep out of the way. They can even produce high-pitched sounds themselves to confuse the bats.

**How good is a moth's nose?**

The male silk moth can detect the scent of a female ready to mate from 7 miles (11 km) away. His "nose" is actually a pair of feathery antennae. These contain the scent receptors.

**What is a silkworm?**

The silkworm is the caterpillar of the mulberry silk moth *Bombyx mori*. Like many other moth larvae, it can make silk threads, but its cocoon is made of incredibly long threads up to ¾ mile (1.2 km) long, ideal for spinning into cloth. Silkworms have been bred in captivity for at least 2,000 years in China.

**Which moth smells like a goat?**

The goat moth has a larva that produces a strong smell of goat. The larva lives inside a tree for three or four years before it is mature. It can be up to 3 in (7.5 cm) long. It can cause serious damage to the tree because it bores through the wood.

# What is the biggest earthworm?

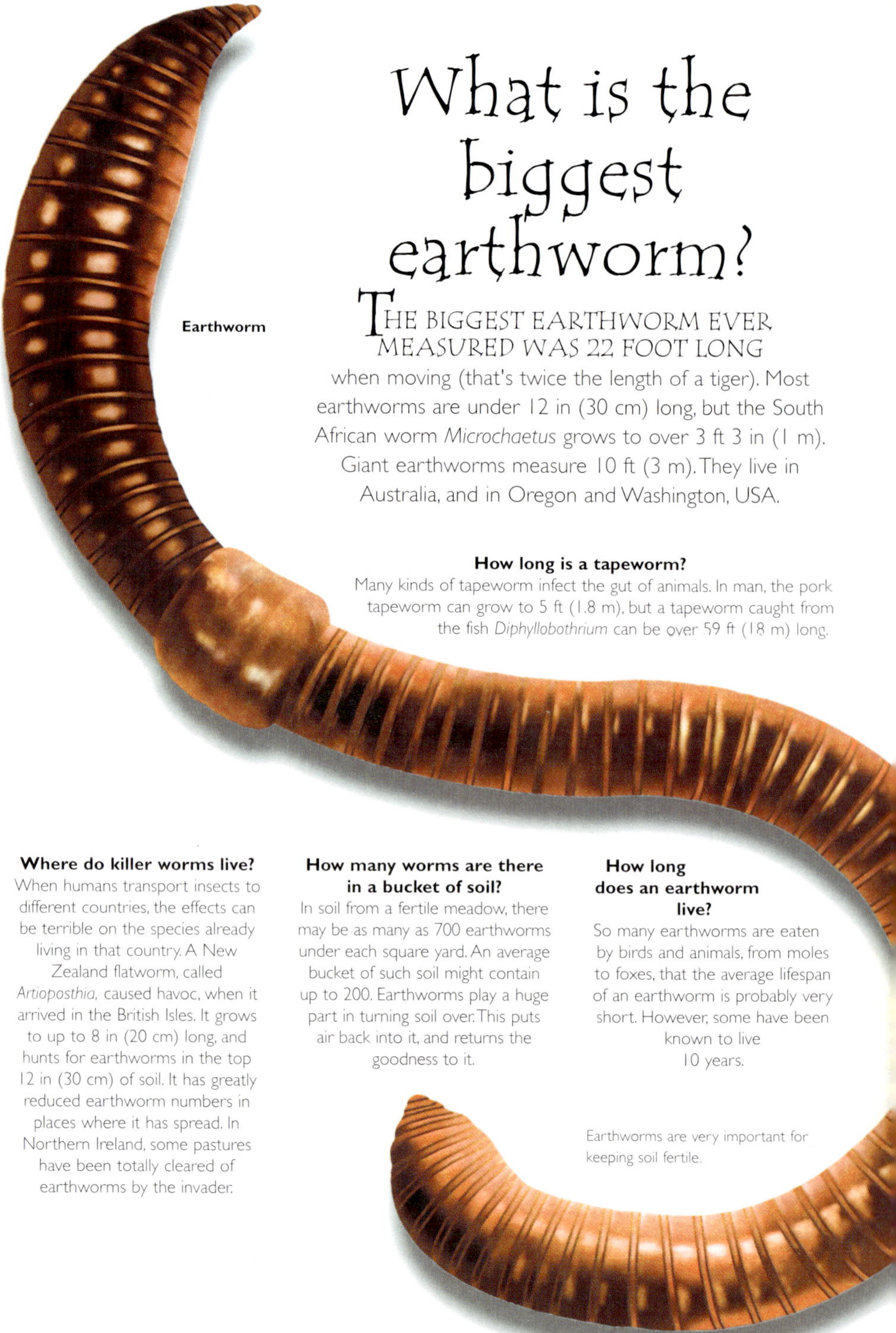

Earthworm

THE BIGGEST EARTHWORM EVER MEASURED WAS 22 FOOT LONG when moving (that's twice the length of a tiger). Most earthworms are under 12 in (30 cm) long, but the South African worm *Microchaetus* grows to over 3 ft 3 in (1 m). Giant earthworms measure 10 ft (3 m). They live in Australia, and in Oregon and Washington, USA.

**How long is a tapeworm?**

Many kinds of tapeworm infect the gut of animals. In man, the pork tapeworm can grow to 5 ft (1.8 m), but a tapeworm caught from the fish *Diphyllobothrium* can be over 59 ft (18 m) long.

**Where do killer worms live?**

When humans transport insects to different countries, the effects can be terrible on the species already living in that country. A New Zealand flatworm, called *Artioposthia*, caused havoc, when it arrived in the British Isles. It grows to up to 8 in (20 cm) long, and hunts for earthworms in the top 12 in (30 cm) of soil. It has greatly reduced earthworm numbers in places where it has spread. In Northern Ireland, some pastures have been totally cleared of earthworms by the invader.

**How many worms are there in a bucket of soil?**

In soil from a fertile meadow, there may be as many as 700 earthworms under each square yard. An average bucket of such soil might contain up to 200. Earthworms play a huge part in turning soil over. This puts air back into it, and returns the goodness to it.

**How long does an earthworm live?**

So many earthworms are eaten by birds and animals, from moles to foxes, that the average lifespan of an earthworm is probably very short. However, some have been known to live 10 years.

Earthworms are very important for keeping soil fertile.

**Do worms eat potatoes?**

Roundworms are shapeless worms with two pointed ends. They are very common. Most are tiny, and live in water or damp soil. You can hold up to 1000 in just one handful. One kind of roundworm, the potato-root eelworm, is a serious pest. It weakens the plant by living in its roots. Other roundworms, such as the hookworm of the southern USA, live inside humans as parasites.

**Which worms can you catch from a dog?**

Dogs often have parasitic worms inside them. These can include a tiny tapeworm called *Echinococcus*. The larva forms a cyst the size of an orange inside the host animal. The worm's eggs are passed out in dog faeces. A dog that has licked itself clean may have eggs on its tongue. If it licks the face or hand of a human, they may be infected. A huge cyst can form in their body, or most deadly of all, in the brain.

**Which worm lives inside people?**

The human blood fluke is the "flatworm" that causes the disease bilharzia, which attacks millions of people in the Middle East and Africa. The larvae of the worms are released into the water, and burrow into the skin of humans who are wading through the water. Pairs of flukes then live in veins in the gut. Their eggs are passed out through the person's bladder, damaging it as they go.

**Why do we cook meat?**

Cooking meat can improve the flavour or tenderness, but it is also very useful for killing parasites, and their eggs and larvae, which might otherwise infect us. If there is a tapeworm in the meat, raw or undercooked beef and pork can infect people.

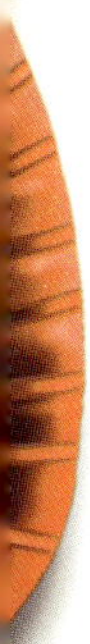

**Leech**

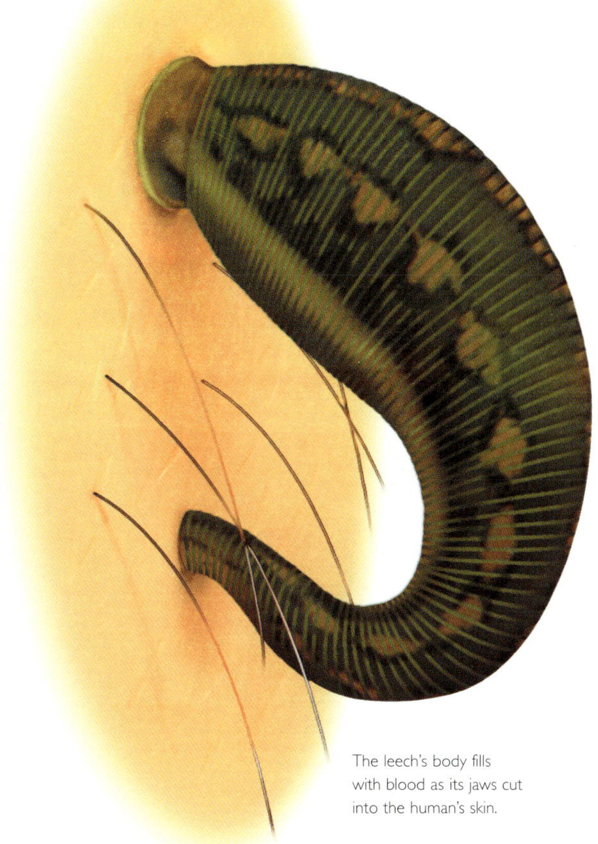

The leech's body fills with blood as its jaws cut into the human's skin.

# Which worm sucks blood?

THE MEDICINAL LEECH SUCKS BLOOD FROM MAMMALS, INCLUDING HUMANS. IN the past, people treated many diseases by "bleeding" the patient. They believed that diseases were caused by too much blood in the body. The leech would use its three teeth to open a wound; its digestive juices anaesthetized wounds and kept blood flowing.

**How big is the biggest snail?**
The shell of the giant African snail Achatina can be up to 13 in (35 cm) long. That is as long as a rabbit. The extended snail is longer. A captive specimen was once measured at 15 in (39 cm) from head to tail, with a shell 10 in long (27 cm), and a weight of 32 oz (900 g).

**Do all snail shells coil the same way?**
In most snails, the shells spiral to the right. If you hold the shell so the mouth is facing you, the mouth is on the right. Some species have a left-handed shell. In each species, all the individuals coil in the same direction.

**How do snails make shells?**
The mantle is a skin that covers the parts of the snail that stay within the shell. The shell substance is produced by the edge of the mantle. The shell has a horny layer, then an inner, strengthening layer of calcium carbonate. This is the same chemical as chalk.

**What do snail eggs look like?**
Some species produce clutches of up to 100, others fewer. In many cases, they are round and transparent, but other species such as the giant African snail have eggs with a hard chalky shell. The eggs are the size of a small bird's egg.

**Giant African snail**

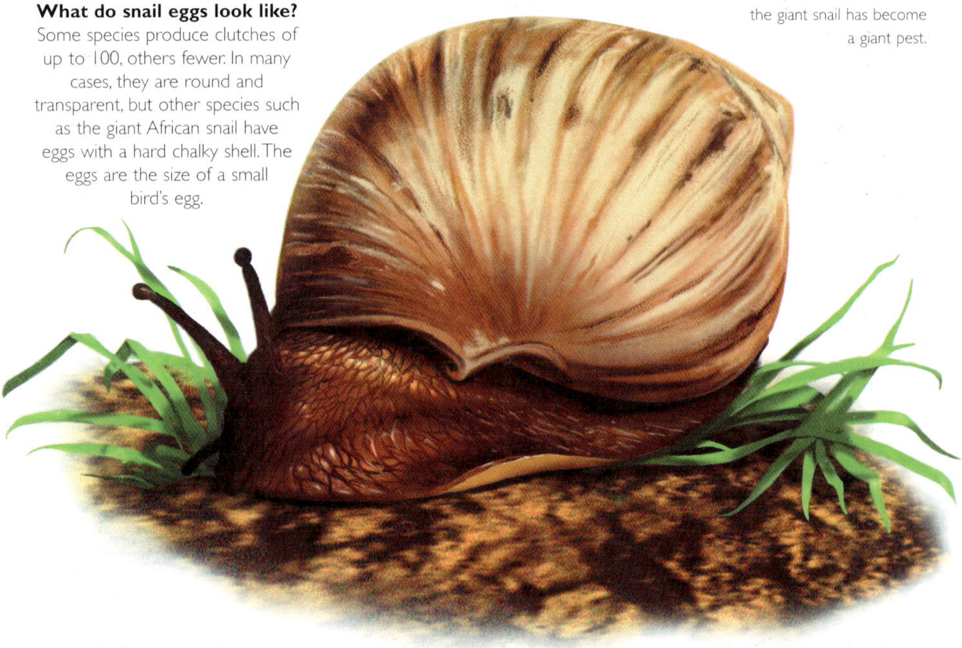

Away from its native land, the giant snail has become a giant pest.

# Which is the world's fastest snail?

MOST SNAILS ARE SO SLOW-MOVING THAT NOBODY HAS BOTHERED TO MEASURE their speed, but the fastest snail on record was an ordinary garden snail *Helix aspersa*. This could move at 0.03 mph (0.05 kph).

**What are the rarest snails in the world?**
The *Partula* snails, of some South Pacific islands, may be the rarest in the world, but they are fighting for survival. Giant African snails were introduced to the islands accidentally, but became a farm pest. So, a meat-eating snail was introduced to control them, but preferred to catch the smaller *Partula* snails, which are ¾ in (2 cm) long. The species is now rare, and it is threatened by habitat loss too, but *Partula* snails are being bred in captivity now, to try and save them.

# Do all slugs eat plants?

MOST SLUGS ARE PLANT-EATERS. SOME ARE pests because they attack our crops, but many prefer to feed on dead or decaying plant matter. Shelled slugs, such as *Testacella,* are unusual because they have a tiny bit of shell left on their backs. They are unusual in another way too; they are meat-eaters. They go underground and chase worms. They harpoon them with their tongues, then suck them into their mouths.

**What do snails do in a drought?**

Although their shells are waterproof, snails' bodies are likely to dry out fast when there is a drought. Most snails are active at night or in wet weather. At other times, they rest in places where water hangs around for a long time. In very dry conditions, many snails make a door for the entrance to their shell. This door, called an epiphragm, is made of a thick layer of dried mucus. A snail can survive for months inside this protection, until damp conditions return.

**Which slugs mate in mid-air?**

Most slugs and snails are both male and female in the same body. Even so, they usually mate with another slug or snail, and mating rituals may be very complicated. For example, one great gray slug meets another on the ground, and starts a slimy embrace. The pair climb up vegetation, entwining and producing so much slime that it forms a rope up to 39 in (1 m) long. The pair dangles from the end of this as they complete their mating in mid-air.

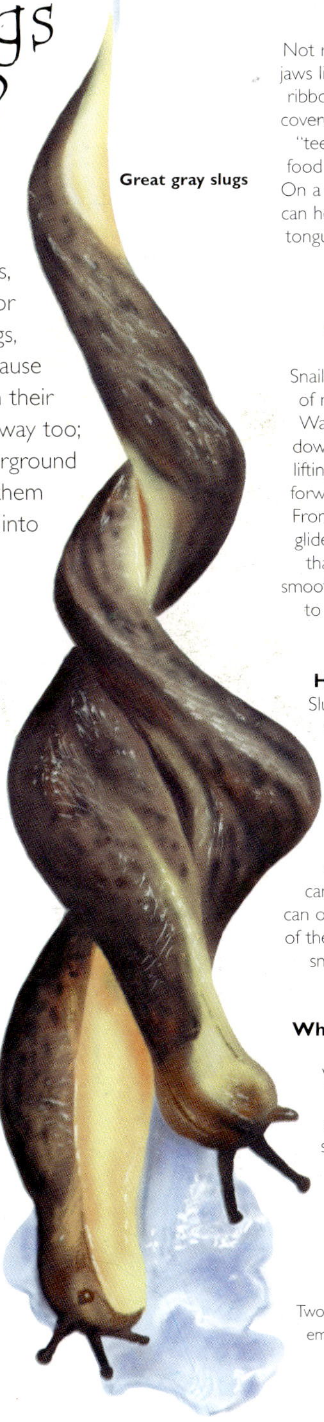

**Great gray slugs**

Two gray slugs mate in a slimy embrace, hanging above the ground.

**Do slugs and snails have teeth?**

Not really. Snails and slugs have no jaws like ours, but they have special ribbon-shaped tongues which are covered in row upon row of horny "teeth." They rasp away at their food and break it into tiny pieces. On a quiet night in the garden, you can hear the noise of snail and slug tongues shredding their food with their file-like tongues.

**How do snails move without legs?**

Snails move on a single thick pad of muscle known as the "foot." Waves of muscle power move down the underside of the foot, lifting sections and moving them forward, as others are put down. From above the snail appears to glide along. The mucus, or slime, that the snail produces, helps smooth its path, and is sticky enough to help it grip when it climbs.

**How do snails breathe?**

Slugs and snails have turned the wall of the mantle (the skin of the snail) into a kind of lung. It is well supplied with blood vessels and encloses a cavity that is full of air. This connects to the outside air through a special hole, that can be opened and closed. You can often see this hole on the right of the body if you look at a slug or snail when it's stretched out.

**Where do slugs hang out in dry weather?**

We always see slugs in wet weather, but where do they go when it dries up? Unlike a snail, a slug cannot hide out in its shell during drought. Many slugs simply burrow deep into the earth and stay there until it is wet again.

# Index


## AB
acacia ants 10
ants 8, 9, 10—11
aphids 11, 17, 22
assassin bugs 16

bed-bugs 17
bees 12, 13, 15, 22
beetles 15, 24—5
bird-eating spiders 4
black garden ants 11
black widow spiders 5
blowflies 23
bluebottles 22
bolas spiders 5
boll weevils 25
bombardier beetles 25
brimstone butterflies 26
bugs 17
bumblebees 12, 13, 22
butterflies 26, 27

## C
carpet beetles 24
centipedes 7
cicadas 16
cinnabar moths 27
cochineal bugs 16
crab spiders 5
crickets 18
cuckoo-spit 17

## DEF
damselflies 15
death-watch beetles 24
desert locusts 19
dragonflies 15
driver ants 11
dung beetles 25
dung flies 22

earthworms 28
emperor moths 27
eyespots 27

fireflies 24
flash coloration 18
flatworms 28, 29
fleas 20, 21
flies 15, 22, 23
flour beetles 24
flukes 29
frog hopper bugs 17
fruit-flies 22
funnel-web spiders 5

## GHI
giant African snails 30
goat moths 27
goliath beetles 24
grasshoppers 18
great gray slugs 31
greenflies 17

hawthorn bugs 17
head lice 21
honeybees 12, 13
hookworms 29
horse-flies 22
house dust mites 7
hoverflies 22

imperial scorpions 6

## JKLM
jiggers 21

ladybirds 24
leaf-cutter ants 10, 11
leeches 29
lice 21
locusts 19
longhorn beetles 24

magnetic termites 9
mantises 14
mating
- ants 11
- beetles 24
- dragonflies 15
- scorpions 6
- slugs 31
- spiders 5

mealworm beetles 24
midges 23
millipedes 7
mites 7
mole crickets 18
monarch butterflies 26
*Morpho* butterflies 26
mosquitoes 22, 23
moths 26, 27
mulberry silk moths 27
museum beetles 24

## NOPQR
nectar 12
nits 21
"no-see-ums" 23

painted ladies 26
pangolins 8
parasites 21, 23, 29
parasitic wasps 13
*Partula* snails 30
peacock butterflies 26
periodical cicadas 16
pork tapeworms 28
potato-root eelworms 29
potter wasps 13
praying mantises 14
protozoa 8

queen bees 12

recluse spiders 5
red admirals 26
rhinoceros beetles 24
roundworms 29
royal jelly 12

## STU
sand wasps 13
saw-footed stick insects 14
sawflies 13
scarab beetles 25
scorpions 6
shield bugs 17
short-horned grasshoppers 18
silk moths 27
silkworms 27
slave-maker ants 10
slugs 31
snails 30, 31
spiders 4—5
stick insects 14, 15
stink bugs 17

tamanduas 8
tapeworms 28, 29
tarantulas 4
termites 8—9
ticks 6, 7
tiger moths 27
tortoiseshell butterflies 26
tropical orb spiders 4
tsetse flies 23
tumbu flies 22

## VWXYZ
vine phylloxera aphids 17

warble flies 22
wasps 12, 22
weevils 24, 25
wolf spiders 4, 5
wood ants 10
wood wasps 13
woolly bears 24
worms 28—9

yucca moths 27